She Seems Fine To Me

She Seems Fine To Me
Behind the Scenes of Birth, Babies and My Broken Brain

Kimberley Nixon

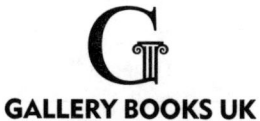
GALLERY BOOKS UK

London · New York · Amsterdam/Antwerp · Sydney/Melbourne · Toronto · New Delhi

First published in Great Britain by Gallery Books, an imprint of Simon & Schuster UK Ltd, 2026

Copyright © Kimberley Nixon, 2026

The right of Kimberley Nixon to be identified as the author of this work has been asserted in accordance with the Copyright, Designs and Patents Act, 1988.

1 3 5 7 9 10 8 6 4 2

Simon & Schuster UK Ltd
1st Floor
222 Gray's Inn Road
London WC1X 8HB

For more than 100 years, Simon & Schuster has championed authors and the stories they create. By respecting the copyright of an author's intellectual property, you enable Simon & Schuster and the author to continue publishing exceptional books for years to come. We thank you for supporting the author's copyright by purchasing an authorised edition of this book.

No amount of this book may be reproduced or stored in any format, nor may it be uploaded to any website, database, language-learning model, or other repository, retrieval, or artificial intelligence system without express permission. All rights reserved. Enquiries may be directed to Simon & Schuster, 222 Gray's Inn Road, London WC1X 8HB or RightsMailbox@simonandschuster.co.uk

www.simonandschuster.co.uk
www.simonandschuster.com.au
www.simonandschuster.co.in

Simon & Schuster Australia, Sydney
Simon & Schuster India, New Delhi

The authorised representative in the EEA is Simon & Schuster Netherlands BV, Herculesplein 96, 3584 AA Utrecht, Netherlands. info@simonandschuster.nl

The author and publishers have made all reasonable efforts to contact copyright-holders for permission, and apologise for any omissions or errors in the form of credits given. Corrections may be made to future printings.

Simon & Schuster strongly believes in freedom of expression and stands against censorship in all its forms. For more information, visit BooksBelong.com.

A CIP catalogue record for this book is available from the British Library

Hardback ISBN: 978-1-3985-5753-6
eBook ISBN: 978-1-3985-5754-3

Typeset in Bembo Std by
Palimpsest Book Production Limited, Falkirk, Stirlingshire

Printed and Bound in the UK using 100% Renewable Electricity
at CPI Group (UK) Ltd

To T, my greatest gift. Thank you for showing me who I was meant to be all along.

To C, the great love of my life. Always my other person on the planet.

To my dad, my greatest cheerleader. Every dog has his day.

And to you, the person so terrified by their own thoughts that you think you won't survive. I'm proof that you can, will and even thrive.

Love always,
Kimbo x

Contents

	Foreword	xi
	Prologue	xv
1	IVF	1
2	A Pregnant Pause	31
3	The Golden Hour	57
4	The Fourth Trimester	79
5	Intrusive Thoughts	105
6	Dear Diary	139
7	All Aboard the Good Relationship	199
8	Who Do You Think You Are?	221
9	The Real Afterbirth	235
	Epilogue	257
	Acknowledgements	263
	Notes	265

Author's Note

This book contains personal accounts of traumatic birth and mental illness, including periods of suicidal ideation. These experiences are shared honestly and may be difficult for some readers.

If you are affected by these passsages, support is available via Samaritans (116 123), NHS 111 or your GP.

Foreword

Professor Lynne M Drummond
Honorary Consultant Psychiatrist, SW London and St George's Mental Health NHS Trust and Visiting Professor, University of Hertfordshire

She Seems Fine to Me is raw, honest and deeply moving. It made me pause, think, wince and even shed a tear – in my opinion, this book should be required reading for anyone working in the healthcare profession.

Most who choose to work in a caring profession do so because they genuinely want to help others and deliver outstanding care to all their patients. Sadly, though, standards of care often fall short, and this can have profound consequences – especially for those who are frightened and unfamiliar with the medical system. Institutional pressures, exhaustion and, at times, a failure to listen – especially to women – can lead to care that feels dismissive or callous.

Sadly, Kimberley's delayed diagnosis came as no surprise to me. While there is now greater public awareness of OCD, it remains widely misunderstood. The term is often casually used to describe someone who is, for example, fastidious or tidy (they might be referred to as 'a little bit OCD'), trivialising what is, in fact, a severe mental health disorder affecting 3 per cent of the population: OCD is recognised by the World Health Organization as one of the leading causes of disability worldwide and carries an elevated risk of suicide.

At the core of OCD are intrusive, unwanted thoughts, images or impulses which are profoundly distressing and often represent the worst possible thing the individual can imagine – harming someone they love, for example. In an effort to calm the terror of the unwanted thoughts and images, OCD sufferers engage in compulsions, which are acts intended to reduce the anxiety caused by the intrusive thoughts. Compulsions may temporarily relieve the anxiety – but usually only briefly, so the cycle continues.

There are effective treatments for OCD. Cognitive Behavioural Therapy (CBT) offers a structured way for OCD sufferers to confront their thoughts without performing compulsions. Medication such as serotonin reuptake inhibiting medicine (SRIs) also works for many patients. Recent studies in the US and the UK have confirmed that people with OCD often suffer for years before receiving the correct treatment.

It probably won't come as much of a surprise when I say that specialist services for pregnant and postpartum women only started to be developed towards the end of the twentieth century – and, historically, the focus has been primarily on psychosis and bipolar disorder. Yet OCD frequently worsens or first appears during pregnancy and particularly after birth. This is devastating for a new mum who expects to feel joy and fulfillment, but instead has to deal with the onset of terrifying intrusive thoughts. Shame and fear of judgement often then prevent women from admitting what they are experiencing.

Pregnancy and childbirth are major life events which involve huge psychological adjustment. They are also times of intense hormonal fluctuation – oestrogen and progesterone (which influence serotonin and GABA systems in the brain) rise during pregnancy and fall sharply after the baby is born. Oxytocin is generally associated with love and bonding, but due to its complex interaction with the brain – and how it intensifies the feeling of responsibility and fear of harm – it can sometimes worsen OCD symptoms. On top of this, levels of cortisol (associated with stress response) are elevated following birth and likely to be exacerbated by worry and lack of sleep. Most mothers feel overwhelmed by the responsibility of caring for a fragile newborn, making this period of time one of extreme vulnerability.

Kim articulates so well the terror of intrusive thoughts and the impact of not being believed or understood. As well as opening up conversations around a topic that is so often shrouded in shame, her story reminds us that perinatal OCD isn't rare and that it is a treatable medical condition.

Stories like Kim's need to be told; they are a vital part of challenging the stigma around perinatal mental health – I admire Kim's courage in choosing to open up and write about her experience. In telling her story, she is helping others to feel less alone; her words show us that there is hope and that recovery is possible. I hope readers will take comfort, that clinicians will take note and that, ultimately, the care given to women experiencing perinatal OCD will improve.

Prologue

I *hate* the word journey.

Although, yes, technically, this is a memoir of my emotional journey through early motherhood, I feel like such a wanker using that word in the emotional, X-Factor sob-story context. So, from this point onwards, I won't be using the J-word, unless I'm talking about a physical expedition or the 1980s rock band (which I can't see coming up, to be honest).

Having said that, I am just a small-town girl living in a lonely world. But we'll get to that.

Right, now I've set the tone for what's to come, turn the page and let's dig deep into my wonderfully, brutally, fucked-up mind.

PS I'm sorry about the swearing – it's just how me and my brain talk to each other. Hop aboard! Next stop: No Filter Junction.

1

IVF

(Or Internal Vagina Fails)

Married? Check. Thirty? Check. Solid career? Check. Well, if you call being a freelance actor solid.

What, then, could be more natural than trying to conceive (or TTC as it's commonly referred to on Mumsnet, a place I would become all-too-familiar with over the next five years). Believe me when I say I could write a dissertation on Mumsnet entitled 'How to Be Passive-Aggressive, Judgemental and Only Mildly Helpful', but that's for another time.

So yes, I was thirty years old, and my husband and I had been together for eleven years, married for one. He's the love of my life, my childhood(ish) sweetheart. Children were always on the cards for us, but more as fluffy kid-shaped outlines somewhere in the distant and rose-tinted future, yet to be filled in. (Strangely, in the first few years of motherhood, my child would appear to me more as scratchy Quentin Blake-esque inked illustrations I was desperate to soften and colour in, but we'll get to that later.)

Like many other women, I'd been on birth control throughout

my twenties – Microgynon, to be precise – originally for severe period pain and bleeding that could last for up to a fortnight, later because getting pregnant at drama school or in the early days of my career would, I was led to believe, be a disaster.

I remember exactly when we started 'trying'. It was Valentine's Day 2016 and I'd booked an impromptu trip to Vienna. I remember it well because I just have one of those brains that remembers random things in shocking detail. I even recall the flight number (EZY608 if you're interested) and the cushioned feel of the mottled brown carpet of our tiny living room beneath my socks, while my husband and I argued about my need for spontaneous endorphin-chasing trips and his total aversion to 'wasting' money.

I've never known two people more perfect for each other, who love each other unconditionally, but who can't go a full half-hour without quarrelling. In today's parlance, bickering would be called our love language, although it's mainly because I like winding him up. And because he's wrong about a lot. Although I will concede he's right about an awful lot more than I care to admit.

Anyway, my husband also isn't fond of flying. It's not a phobia, but he doesn't enjoy the thought of the flight, specifically take-off and landing. For over twenty years, since our first holiday together to Italy in 2005, I have always reached out and grabbed his hand during those turbulent moments. I'm the holiday planner of the wider family, the one who gets excited about going away. I book all the flights, transfers and villas for big family get-aways. My brother-in-law jokingly calls me Nixon Travel. I enjoy it. The organisation side and just having something to look forward to. It means real life is on hold for a while and, as you'll find out, I generally find life to be quite overwhelming. I think it's partly why I love Christmas. It's this sacred time and space where everything is suspended for a while; no one can pester you about work, or school, or college because . . . it's Christmas. It's a protected time. Ring-fenced reassurance. We'll sort that after Christmas. Need something? Is after Christmas okay? It's a relief to feel the communal pressure's off for a few days – along with everyone else because usually it feels like it's just me who constantly craves that. It's probably why I find January so soul-suckingly oppressive: I'm skint, it's dark at 3pm and all my 'do that after Christmases' are coming home to roost. I have two settings: right this minute or push, push, push it back.

Anyway, flying aside, my husband also doesn't like spending money. Sometimes I think he believes anything outside the basics of food and drink (and plants! He's a gardener) is a frivolity. But that may be his strong Welsh frugal roots coming into play. Put flying and spending money together and you have a European mini-break that he groans and grumbles about until we're on the second day of the holiday, when finally he loves it. Hence, our argument. Not the most romantic precursor to our trip or starting a family.

We traipsed around Austria's capital, my history-loving husband explaining the city's complex background and shaking his head at me for wondering aloud whether Hitler or Freud had ever sat in my chair at lunch.

I was already away with the fairies planning for a Christmas baby. He tried to manage my expectations – 'it's unlikely to work on the first go' – but I'm very much a black-and-white thinker and, since I'd taken the monumental decision to stop taking the pill and become a mother – even though childbirth had terrified me from a young age, after I'd heard the fun factoid that you were supposed to push something the size of a melon through something the size of a lemon – I felt the universe should get with the programme.

'Ooh, maybe we could call her Vienna if it's a girl?'

'So everyone will know where we did it? Like the Beckhams?' he threw back incredulously.

Okay, maybe not. But it would still be lovely. This time next year, I thought, we'll be parents.

★

You're probably way ahead of my naïve, broody little self in realising it didn't work the first time, or the hundreds of times after that as we failed to 'catch' (God, Mumsnet is gross) over the next four years. Having felt pretty smug that I'd successfully managed to not get pregnant before my wedding at twenty-nine years of age, the cruel irony that I would then spend the first half of my thirties desperately trying to have a baby and mourning every period was certainly not lost on me. Fertility apps and reproductive windows soon entered the picture and suddenly, what was once an idealistic endeavour born of love and the desire to start our own little family, became scheduled sex and invasive testing.

According to NHS guidelines, you should try naturally for one year. We did. It was fun; we were still young and hopeful that next time would be the charm. We tried, tried and tried again. A love-song mix on in the background trying to keep the romance aspect alive – playing the same ten songs (this need for familiarity and repetition will come up later). I would lie with my legs in the air, post-coitally, for good measure, and

IVF

to this day I can't hear Roberta Flack's 'First Time Ever I Saw Your Face' without getting phantom pins and needles in my feet. Each month we'd patiently wait to see if that telltale spot of blood would appear. Predictably, it always did, so it was time for some investigative testing to see why we weren't getting that BFP (Big Fat Positive – again, Mumsnet).

One small problem with the NHS is that everything takes so long. You call your GP, your appointment is a fortnight away, you attend, they refer, it then takes another six weeks for the next slot with whatever specialist to arrive by post and it turns out that that consultation isn't for another two months anyway. You finally go to the fated appointment; you either have something put in you or leave some kind of deposit behind. You wait six to eight weeks for the results – luckily all clear for us – and you're told to head back to your GP. Then the merry dance starts once more and this time the referral is for yet another embarrassing test at some far-off date in the future. So, with everything from blood tests to gauge hormone levels (such as progesterone or gonadotropins), pelvic ultrasounds to assess reproductive organs and STI screenings for the woman, to multiple semen analyses for the men, it's very easy for a year or two to slip by, on top of the original year of trying naturally.

Our lives became punctuated by fertility appointments; all the while we were trying to have meaningful sex that was slowly becoming more mechanical and a tad resentful. By the nature of the timetable, you must go by the woman's cycle. The woman has to keep track and said woman with vagina and womb has to tell the man with the penis 'we should do it now'. Not because you feel like it, not when the mood takes you, but by huffily pointing to a calendar on a fucking fertility app because it says it's your 'fertile window'. The phrase 'I don't care if you don't feel like it' or 'do you want a baby or not?' definitely came up on our Barren Bonking Bingo Card more than once. House!

*

Then one day, it's decided you should be put on The List. IVF, shit. The Big One. Well, I thought, I'd definitely get pregnant now, because all I'd heard was how someone's cousin's boss's daughter had tried for years and then, as soon as they went for IVF, she naturally fell pregnant. Oh, well, brilliant. Forget planning sex around my cycle; his sperm and my egg would somehow intuit that the pressure was off. Reverse psychology. Meet up in the fallopian tube, guys, see if we care!

Out of desperation, I invested heavily in The App. I'd religiously put a little heart in the calendar when we had sex and add the little blood drop icon when I had a period. I was like some mad, nymphomaniacal data collector. But even I absolutely drew the fucking line at labelling my vaginal discharge from a disgusting drop-down menu of descriptions such as 'creamy and cloudy' or 'thick and stretchy' to finally 'raw egg whites'. Fuck. Off.

I knew about growing a human being from scratch inside my body; I was aware of the pain of childbirth and I'd even got my head around the fact that, at some point, I was expected to have fully functioning udders. But in no film, book or TV show that I'd ever seen depicting this whole experience, was I supposed to define the consistency of my luteal phase output. No, thank you.

My husband, meanwhile, had to jizz in a cup. This was, apparently, comparable in the embarrassment stakes to me having

IVF

my legs spread in stirrups in an operating theatre while a long plastic straw was inserted into my vagina to allow a special dye to be pumped into the ovaries to check for blockages. It was humiliating, uncomfortable and certainly not as fun as orgasming into a sample bottle. Then to top it off, with my head laid back on the starched hospital pillow, I heard the nurse suddenly chirp up, 'Were you in *Cranford*?'

★

I was indeed in *Cranford*. But very much like my route into motherhood, my acting career wasn't exactly arrived at conventionally. I'm not from one of those 'acting families'; I dreamt of being even distant cousins with the 'connected'. In fact, I was raised in a small village called Ynysybwl two miles outside the Valleys town of Pontypridd in South Wales. I was actually born in Bristol in 1985 to Welsh parents, who spent a couple of years across the border in England for my dad's job but we moved back to Wales when I was four years old, so I spent the Nineties and Noughties – formative years – here in Ponty. This makes me a millennial. We're the last generation to remember house phones: the age-group who get anxiety if our mobile buzzes with an unknown number and who, no matter how hard we try, can't let go of trainer socks. I am also the only girl in a family of seven children. Don't do the maths – I have six brothers.

I worked hard in school and, for much of my childhood, tried to be what you might call 'a good girl'. With so much male energy in the house, I felt the weight of being the only girl. The polite young lady. Well behaved. Even though my brain was quietly on fire and I wanted to wear jeans, not dresses, and climb trees as well as play with dolls. It felt like saying no was a big . . . no-no. It made you 'difficult' or a 'little madam'. It was impolite to not bend to other people's needs or schedules and so just as you pour hot liquid jelly into novelty moulds, I set into a wibbly-wobbly people-pleasing peacemaker.

I went to a state school of about a thousand kids in Cilfynydd (Kil-VUN-ithe). Coedylan Comprehensive Upper School was built on the site of a coal-mining disaster that killed 290 men and boys, as well as 123 horses, in 1894 – so that felt like a good omen. The school tie of Coedylan was a vivid Cadbury's purple with a red and white stripe. Your level of coolness directly correlated to how short you wore that tie in the late Nineties/ early Noughties. Needless to say, my tie was worn to the regulation length like a good girl, unlike the character I'd come to play in the now-cult film *Angus, Thongs and Perfect Snogging*. My schoolfriends howled when, after *Cranford*, I was cast as Slaggy Lindsay. Low-cut tops, thick stumpy tie and lip-gloss? At school? I had *never* been that cool.

I wanted to do well, but more importantly, I *needed* to do well. We were from a working-class ex-mining town but my dad had a good job as a regional manager for an oil company, often on the road. With nine mouths to feed, we always had everything we could ever need but knew the true value of things. I was under no illusions that my only way out was through my education. The more qualified I became, the more self-sufficient and financially independent my future self would be and the less I'd have to rely on other people to do whatever I wanted. These were quite big ideals for a frizzy-haired, pale eleven-year-old unknowingly riddled with intrusive thoughts and repetitive thought loops. I secretly hoped I was bound for a special, maybe even supernatural fate. Like Buffy or Sabrina.

It's ironic that I never did leave my hometown, continuing to live here until this very day and loving my life because of it.

Looking back, the absolute and mindboggling scale of self-absorption when you're a teenager is both staggering and strangely comforting. Your world is so small but there's the promise of a bigger, brighter one, right around the corner. I remember watching the news, in my typically early-2000s lilac and blue bedroom, of the planes hitting the Twin Towers and writing in my diary about how mean this boy was being to me, even though everyone said it was just because he liked me. This colossal, earth-shattering, devastating geo-political event was playing out before my eyes, but it wasn't as important as my pubescent poetry (which was far too complicated for anyone else to grasp. Like, you just wouldn't get it. I was feeling things no other human being in existence has ever felt – duh!). Weirdly, I find that quite reassuring. It's evidence that you live in a safe part of the world and war and famine are just things on the telly.

I studied, I overcompensated and I strived when things didn't always come naturally (maths). Now, I'm probably held up as a successful alumnus who's remembered for being quiet, polite and diligent. While that's lovely, it's not exactly true. I was chock-full of anxiety and self-doubt the entire time. I found friendships, especially females ones, difficult to navigate. Boys, I got. They tended to swear or punch out their frustration and once expelled, it was forgotten. Girls had this whole new level of passive–aggressive subtle behaviours that I would study and try to replicate. I was different, it seemed, from the start. But I hated confrontation and conforming helped avoid that. Later, with a hugely atheist boyfriend (now husband) and a devoted Christian for a best friend in Jess (you'll hear more about her later), lively debates between them would leave me frazzled in the middle. It's funny to think of it now, as we're all too fucking tired and wrapped up in our kids to care about silly arguments and we just laugh about how carefree and rich with time and energy we used to be. I'm not saying there isn't any merit in raising a considerate young woman who thinks of others and is eager to help, but when her self-worth becomes inextricably connected to how useful others deem her to be, over a long period of time, it can become a big problem.

While I worried that I was unusual or broken, I hoped that this was just the first act of my hero arc. Surely I would push through this near-constant feeling of alienation, this sense of not quite being like everyone else, until some wise old sage stepped from the shadows, spouting worthy exposition about my great destiny. That it wasn't that I was odd or didn't belong – I was simply in the wrong place. It wasn't my time until now, when the world needed me. That hasn't happened yet, by the way, but if I am slated to be the next saviour of mankind, they'd better get a shift on, as my back is only getting worse.

So, while it's technically true that I was a high-achieving pupil who went on to star in television, stage and film productions, eventually winning a BAFTA (the old Ricky Gervais joke from *Extras* of it only being a Welsh one tickling my brain stem), not many people know of the fretfulness, disquiet and sadness that accompanied much of my schooldays. I always felt on the back foot, was constantly misreading social situations – which, as we all know, at that age is tantamount to teenage harakiri – and cried a lot, alone at home, because I just didn't understand why I couldn't be like everyone else, carefree and enjoying my youth. I didn't get why a lower grade hit me so hard, or why I would seize up if a boy showed any interest in me (because what if I was a rubbish kisser or had bad breath and he told everyone, and my life was ruined?). No, better to keep to myself. However, these preoccupations weren't just superficial, they went deeper than I could possibly comprehend – and wouldn't until nearly twenty years later.

When it became time to decide on a university, I duly used five of my six options to apply to good, solid institutions to gain a good, solid degree. I thought I'd become a teacher or a journalist, maybe a lawyer. But I did some work experience with a news outlet in Cardiff and, as I sat shadowing a journalist on the court's press bench, I couldn't quite get my head around why they were taking no notes for the horrendous case of child abuse being heard but scribbled like crazy when a Welsh beauty queen was in the dock for assaulting someone at a nightclub. Apparently, the former story was too depressing and people didn't want to read about it. Wasn't it more important, though? Maybe mainstream journalism wasn't for me.

I did have a long-held yet fanciful dream though. I wanted to become an actress. Although I'd been involved in a lot of drama including performing and being behind the scenes in school productions, I'd never confided this to anyone. I would watch movies in my bedroom and rewind my favourite bits of dialogue, mouthing along with the actor on screen. For those few seconds, I could be someone other than myself and the freedom of that was intoxicating. True escapism. Unbeknownst to anyone but me and my dad – whom I consider to be one of my best friends (we've established I'm a loser) – I submitted an application to the Royal Welsh College of Music and Drama (RWCMD) and bagged an audition. The problem was, I had no idea whatsoever how to audition for anything. This was pre-YouTube days and you couldn't just watch a tutorial online. And, since I was so certain I wouldn't get in and this was all a ridiculous pipe dream, I couldn't really ask anyone for help or guidance, either.

I needed to prepare two monologues – one Shakespearean, one contemporary – and a song. Oh god, a song. Singing was not a strength of mine. I could barely sing in public without turning into a beetroot. I decided to basically mimic Renée Zellweger as Roxy Hart in *Chicago* and thought my best bet was to think of it as an acting exercise rather than a demonstration of my musicality. That seemed to make it less daunting. But what about the actual format of this audition – did you start with pleasantries or just walk into the room and burst into a soliloquy? I'd just have to wing it.

I fell into the trap that most young performers do, thinking that the audition is a test of your memory rather than what it really is: a performance, an emotional connection to the story. I didn't sleep for a week, running my speeches over and over in my mind. My automatic, repetitive tendencies came up trumps here. I can't remember what I wore but I do know I worried endlessly about it.

On the day itself, my dad wished me luck as he dropped me at the RWCMD building on North Road in Cardiff, and I took some deep breaths to try to steady my nerves. Walking into the reception area, I was hit by a wall of sound: thirty people practising their monologues. Everyone seemed to be from London and have oodles of confidence. This was their third or fourth audition for a drama school. How many had I applied to? 'Oh, just this one'. This was often met with pitying looks from seasoned auditionees. The odds were not in my favour. The truth was, I needed to stay close to home for family reasons. These reasons were long and varied and probably deserving of their own book, but also by being a Welsh student at a Welsh conservatoire, I would get a reduced rate in my tuition. I simply couldn't have afforded to attend a drama school in London even if I had managed to pay all the audition fees and got in.

I quickly discovered that we were being divided into groups of ten to audition. Holy shit. So not only did I have to perform outside of my bedroom to a panel of judges, but I had to do it in front of nine other judgemental hopefuls. We were escorted into a room I would come to know well over the next three years as a rehearsal space – a small, rectangular room with varnished wooden floors, windows along one side and a mirrored wall along the other. There was no hiding when you could see yourself as well as doubles of everyone else. Five candidates sat along the windows and five along the mirrors. I was on the window side, so I could see myself growing scarlet in real time. Excellent.

Behind the table at the head of the room sat four or five adults. I can't remember them exactly, but I know Dave Bond, the college's Head of Acting, was there and an actress named Nicola Reynolds, who I recognised from the TV show *Ideal* with Johnny Vegas. I would later work with Johnny in one of those full circle moments that sometimes sweep past you in life.

As your name was called, you had to stand in the centre of this mirrored chamber and deliver your monologue. You could choose whether to start with a Shakespearean or contemporary piece. I'd decided on Emilia's speech from *Othello*, as I knew the play inside out from A-Level English and thought it probably a bit too obvious to have yet another innocent-looking blonde play Desdemona. This part had a bit more guts, a bitterness that I thought they perhaps wouldn't expect from me. I was right.

My contemporary speech was from *Equus* by Peter Schaffer, which, if you haven't seen it, is ostensibly a play about a boy who maybe wants to have sex with a horse. I decided to play his mother (someone who would have been at least twenty-five years my senior at the time) and almost, *almost*, went down the route of playing the hunched, croaky-voiced, talc-in-the-hair 'old lady', but pulled back just in time. I was playing the mother of a mentally ill teenage son and had absolutely no idea what I was talking about.

With these two texts simmering around my nervous mind, my name was called. I went to stand in the middle of this room, with my peers and experienced actors and tutors staring at me from behind their *X-Factor* grey table. I'd dragged my plastic chair into the centre with me; there was a low murmur in the room that this was a risky move. Or was I an avant-garde genius? Time would tell. I did my pieces, got the words right and almost, *almost* enjoyed it at points before then scurrying back to the safety of the group once I'd finished.

Eventually, all ten of us had completed our auditions. Some went better than others, some were smiling, some looked disappointed. We were thanked for our time and asked if the following could stay behind for the musical audition. The others would be dismissed, but they stressed this had no bearing on the outcome of whether you'd be successful in the end. Hmm, that smelt very faintly of bullshit, we thought collectively.

'Kimberley Nixon.'

Shit, were they calling out the people who were staying or those who could leave? Judging by the sad trudge of the people not called, a spark of hope ignited deep in my belly.

YES! I'd made it through. I could hardly believe it.

SHIT, I'd made it through. Now I had to sing.

I spent the next half an hour with my jaw on the floor due to the phenomenal musical talent of the others. Their voices were rich and creamy, confident and powerful. I knew this was a bad idea. What was I thinking? Oh well, in for a penny. It was my turn. I stood in the central spot once more and launched into 'Nowadays' by Roxie Hart.

I channelled (read: copied) Renée and even recreated her low-key dance routine. Lord, help me. I was certainly, let's call it *brave*, shall we?

My heart was beating so rapidly I worried I'd just keel over, but I imagined myself valiantly continuing to do the punctuated finger clicks, Bob Fosse-style, while lying prostrate on the shiny, worn wooden floor, being dragged out but simply refusing to let the dream die.

I didn't fall over or spontaneously combust. There weren't any boos and jeers, but there certainly wasn't a standing ovation either. That's it, I was done. I'd done it. I'd auditioned for drama school. We filed out, all relieved it was finally over, and as I passed by Dave Bond, he mused, 'You look like Amanda Holden.' I smiled and replied, 'Oh, fuck off', and he chuckled. As soon as I rounded the doorframe into the corridor my smile dropped. I couldn't believe I'd just said that. To a teacher! I just told the Head of Acting at the Royal Welsh College of Music and Drama to fuck off. It was so unlike me. Brilliant time to come out of your shell, Kim. Well, that was that, then. Only that wasn't that then. Worst spoiler alert ever – I got in. I had to return for a recall where they made me do those speeches again while tidying the room, a standard audition tactic. I didn't have to sing again, thank baby Jesus, but I did have to take part in a group movement class, which was fine. I'd seen MTV – I could blag that. My biggest tips to wannabe acting students is that they're looking for potential and a willingness to give it a go, not perfection or a flawless Britney-with-a-snake routine. Although I could have delivered that if pushed. Probably.

And so, I attended the Royal Welsh College of Music and Drama and received a BA Hons in Acting. Then I found an agent and started to make my way through the murky yet exciting world of the entertainment industry – with no connections and no generational wealth to fall back on. It was through this agent that I landed the role in *Cranford*. There I was, not quite graduated, yet somehow on a film set in a bonnet next to Dame Judi Dench, Imelda Staunton, Michael Gambon and Julia McKenzie. It was an incredible experience; it set the foundations of my career and provided a technical learning curve I would carry with me over the next nineteen years.

Not only this, but the cast and crew were incredibly kind to me, often explaining on-set jargon I hadn't heard before and welcoming my wide-eyed family on set to peek behind the curtain. Remember we had no connection to the entertainment industry at all and this world was completely alien to us. It wasn't a question of pinching myself to check it was real, more like punching myself in the face. I did quickly learn not to bring Valleys folk to a film unit catering van. Red rag to a bull.

But back to that sterile hospital theatre, legs akimbo. When the nurse asked 'were you in *Cranford*?' it was an incredibly easy yet loaded question to answer – but not when eye to whispering eye with my vagina. It all seemed a lifetime ago anyway. All I cared about now was what I'd been trying to prevent for most of my adult life: becoming a mum.

Except, that wasn't quite happening. It turned out my ovaries weren't blocked, but something was preventing me from getting pregnant. They just had to find out what it was. So, the testing continued. I did several jobs in this period, not least *Ordinary Lies* for which I won a Bafta Cymru (but I think it was more for acting with a fringe that didn't suit me than anything else). We didn't tell anyone what was going on, except my best friend, Jess.

Jess and I tell each other everything. We met in Year Seven and bonded over our love of *Pride and Prejudice* (the 1995 BBC TV adaptation, NOT the 2005 film). At the *Cranford* screening, I wandered out of the ladies and bumped into Colin Firth. Just standing there.

'Mr Darcy,' I whispered and, mortified that he'd heard, swivelled on the ball of my foot and ran back into the toilets to immediately text Jess: 'I just called Colin Firth, Mr. Darcy!!!!!!' She talked me down and I went back into the swanky Mayfair cinema. (I later filmed *Easy Virtue* with Colin but unfortunately playing his daughter not his lover). There's something about Jess and I that means we just instinctively get each other. As an example, one Christmas, she arrived at my house for a festive shindig and, upon opening the door, blurted out that she thought she was pregnant.

'Oh my God,' I said, countering with my own news, 'I think I've got a zit on my clit.'

We congratulated one another, no further questioning required, and the merriment of the evening commenced. (I think mine was an ingrowing hair, by the way. Hers, definitely a baby.)

*

The trouble was, Jess wasn't the only one having a baby. In fact, everyone around us was having babies, which meant we were constantly being asked when we were going to start a family. I was starting to think that this whole thing just wasn't fun anymore. Not only that, but it was also causing upset, resentment and an underlying sadness – maybe it just wasn't meant to be.

We had to have a few frank conversations together as a couple during this time. Would 'we' be enough? No kids, just the two of us? That was an easy yes. It would be a different kind of a life, but a good life. We just needed to alter our instinctive reactions to the online baby announcements of friends and family. We concluded that there wasn't a finite number of babies – they got one when we didn't. We weren't fighting over the last turkey in the shop in a mad Christmas Eve dash. That was their baby, their happiness and it truly had nothing to do with us. We were just happy that someone else was getting that moment of joy.

That didn't mean it was always easy to keep the hope alive, until one day my husband said to me bluntly, 'In ten years, we will have kids. I don't know how or what route we'll take, but we'll have children.' He was right – there was no doubt in my mind. We would keep hoping it would happen naturally; we'd crawl along on the NHS IVF waiting list and we'd explore other options, such as adoption. We knew this could be fulfilling – Jess had adopted two boys before she had two biological sons. The love she shared with all of them was unwavering and it didn't make a blind bit of difference how they got there; they were all just one happy family.

This new approach, this new way of thinking, shook everything up. Suddenly every period wasn't a lost opportunity but a bonus month of lie-ins, date nights and watching the entire first series of *The Vampire Diaries* in one night because the whim took me. I could read all day and meet girlfriends for drinks in the evening; he had time to paint and shout at the telly during *Question Time*.

My husband is a bit like the eponymous Beast from the Disney film: gruff, grouchy and, in the winter, he literally walks around the house with a blanket around his shoulders like a cape. It makes me laugh. He is also an exquisite painter, especially portraits, an incredibly knowledgeable gardener and a walking encyclopaedia regarding history, geography, politics and Eighties action films. We were going to be okay.

The other tactic we employed was to name that month's egg something dreadful with the proviso being if that were the one to get fertilised and lead to a pregnancy, we HAD to name the baby that, regardless of sex. So, when my menstrual friend would drop by a few weeks later, it was actually a relief that I wouldn't have a daughter named Tiberius. Or a son called Hortensia. We felt lighter about the whole thing in general.

Hopes were raised several times over the years. A late period here and there, and even a chemical pregnancy (a very early pregnancy loss that occurs just after the embryo has embedded). And while sad, rather than depress us, it just showed me that I could actually *get* pregnant after years of nothing. We would chalk it up to a cosmic win.

The embarrassing medical procedures in the name of finding out what was wrong didn't let up and my husband's humiliation knew no bounds, with having to get his 'sample' to the clinic within a half-hour period to ensure testing viability. He had an absolutely hilarious aversion to using 'The Room', the private part of the IVF clinic set aside to allow male patients to produce their sample for testing. He would rather, say, leave me waiting on a grassy knoll in the middle of an industrial estate, then come back ten minutes later, a bit red-faced, telling me to ask no questions. Barely concealing a smile, I'd get back into the car, and he'd scarcely pulled away from the kerb before I burst out laughing at him. Driving to the hospital, the specimen bottle under his arm for incubation purposes, he mumbled an embarrassed 'oh, fuck off'. I laughed harder.

On another occasion, he disappeared into an empty toilet at the hospital. There wasn't a soul in sight and, hoping to have five minutes alone, he locked himself in the furthest cubicle. He was psyching himself up to do the deed when he heard the squeaky wheels of an IV drip and the soft-slippered shuffle of an elderly gent, who parked up in the stall next to my husband and proceeded to do 'one of the worst shits I've ever heard', according to my mortified spouse.

★

Then, finally, one day, a lady from Wales Fertility Clinic called to tell me it was time. It was our turn. What? It couldn't be. It was, she assured me. We could start IVF treatment the following week and technically be pregnant within the month. Holy shit. I knew it had been four years, but suddenly I wasn't sure I was ready.

We chose to do a particular form of IVF called ICSI – or, to give it its proper name, Intracytoplasmic Sperm Injection. This basically means that they take a single sperm – presumably with tiny tweezers? – and place it into the egg, allowing fertilisation to happen (as opposed to regular IVF, where they just put a load of sperm and eggs in a petri dish and play some

Barry White). Once the embryo is created, it can be transferred back into the uterus and, with the help of a cocktail of drugs, nature would hopefully take its course.

IVF can very generally be summed up into three parts:

Phase One: The Down Regulation

This is where you try to temporarily suppress your natural menstrual cycle and egg production. You put the ovaries 'to sleep' before stimulating them with hormones, so that the following month's egg yield will be higher. Down regulation essentially stops you releasing your eggs before they can be retrieved and then, using gonadotropins, pushes the follicles (which hold the ova) to release more than normal. The follicles on the ultrasound screen always reminded me of waving sea grass. It's a daily regimen of injections to your abdomen. This part really wasn't as bad as I had feared as, with a pinch of belly fat and a glass of Prosecco, I hardly felt it. Yep, that's right: a glass of fizz in one hand, IVF needle in the other – the most middle-class, millennial photograph of my life.

The bit I did struggle with was the internal scans every other day. These are needed to check that your follicles are growing sufficiently and not at risk of developing Ovarian Hyper Stimulation Syndrome (OHSS). This is where the ovaries become enlarged, releasing chemicals that cause blood vessels to leak fluid into the abdomen, causing bloating, abdominal pain and nausea. In severe cases it can become very dangerous, leading to kidney/liver issues, breathing problems and blood clots. The scans are performed with a vaginal wand but, let me tell you, there's nothing magical about it. I'd always been squeamish about anything like this; even tampons were uncomfortable and stressed me out, probably because no one had really explained them to me. I grew up surrounded by boys, after all, and the 'how to' diagram in the instruction leaflet made me light-headed. Was I supposed to chase my finger up there after it? As a girl who got her first period on Christmas Eve, and was told it was a 'gift from Father Christmas', I wasn't pushing anything up anywhere. I'd stick to the pads, thanks. I didn't really change my mindset for the next twenty years, but it turned out I just hadn't been inserting them correctly; I'd assumed no one else could sit down with a tampon half sticking out either. I discovered the error of my ways from an aghast yet bemused Jess.

I'd also put off smear tests for years. I would attend the appointment petrified and with the best will in the world wouldn't allow the nurse to insert the plastic duck beak – sorry, speculum. My mind wanted to allow it but my body would just seize up. A nurse once gruffly asked me if I had sex with my boyfriend. I replied that I did; a terse 'this is no different' was the only reply. I beg to differ, starting with the lighting. It was while doing IVF I would learn of my vaginismus, an involuntary tightening of the muscles in the vagina when something is inserted. It can be humiliating and make simple things like tampons, smear tests and sex daunting. But then I read that Jade Goody had died of cervical cancer that had spread to her bowel, liver and groin at the age of twenty-seven. I haven't missed an appointment since. It's like anything else – practice makes perfect.

The probe of the scan was uncomfortable rather than painful, however, and while I couldn't help tensing up, I knew the internal scans were important. I had to overcome this phobia of mine. In the end, I practised at home with a dildo. Needs must. When I said practice makes perfect, I wasn't just waxing lyrical. This is obviously an embarrassing detail but it's so common and, like a lot of what's to come in this book, not talked about, which leads to shame and embarrassment and that leads to dead women. Rates of vaginismus in women are generally low. It affects 1-6 per cent of women, which can soar in a clinical setting to 30 per cent and a greater 42% in a specialised clinical settings for gynaecological or sexual disorders[1] It's difficult to measure exact numbers of people affected due to factors like embarrassment, stigma or simply the lack of knowledge that what they're experiencing is even a condition. A smear test can save your life. Having a healthy sex life can be integral to a healthy relationship. IVF for an infertile couple who desperately want a child can be life-changing. So I won't be shamed for my dildo practice sessions!

Phase Two: The Egg Collection

No, not a terrible Stephen King thriller, but the process whereby they retrieve this bumper crop of eggs you've been growing for the past couple of weeks. You go into the clinic and, after sedation, they collect the eggs just as the would-be father toddles off to jizz in another cup. My husband had the gall to look put out by this as I was being wheeled into an operating theatre, for fuck's sake. Then (and I'm not clinically trained but), they jab a sperm into an egg and so begins the waiting game to see if it develops into an embryo. I was incredibly lucky to have a bumper crop – they collected thirteen eggs from me which they would individually fertilise and monitor over the next five days. After this I would get a daily call from an anonymous lab technician informing me how they were developing and/or surviving.

You're sedated for egg collection, and as I was coming round from the sedation, still feeling drunk and imploring my husband to 'get up on the hospital bed with me for a cwtch (a welsh word meaning 'cuddle'), the nurses won't mind', I realised said nurses were giggling. It turned out I'd had lots to say while I was under.

'You mean I wasn't asleep?' I asked, aghast.

'No,' the nurse laughed. 'You were telling us all how much your husband likes American Civil War history and how you don't want to ever work in finance.'

I blushed, having no memory of that. All hope that I'd gracefully slipped under and been the perfect patient quickly fell away. Apparently, I kept calling the anaesthetist 'my lovely magic man', too. I gathered it was probably time to leave, but the nurse smiled and reminded me that I needed to eat and drink before I could be discharged. I found it hilarious that I'd brought an egg mayonnaise sandwich with me. My husband rolled his eyes.

Over the next five days, we received daily updates about how our little guys were doing. On day one, we were told that only seven of the thirteen eggs had been successfully fertilised, while the following day they informed us we'd lost another one overnight. By day five, the blastocysts they'd created would need to be of sufficient quality to be transferred into the womb successfully.

There are two types of transfers. Just like your supermarket Christmas turkey, you can choose from fresh or frozen. A fresh transfer means that if five days after your egg retrieval, a viable embryo is good to go, you head back to hospital and have it reinserted. Back up the chute, so to speak. While the lab has been hard at work, you've been taking all the correct hormones to ensure your body is essentially five days pregnant, so the five-day-old blastocyst transfers to the perfect environment, allowing it to embed and the pregnancy to develop. We chose the second option, though – the frozen transfer. This can be for many reasons, but for us it was because I was at risk of developing that nasty condition, OHSS, so it was decided it wouldn't be a very good idea to pump my already swollen ovaries with more drugs. Better to allow my body to have a little breather, with the added bonus that we could also save our frozen embryos for another round of IVF in the future. When the call came through, we were ready to ask the all-important question: did we have anything to freeze?

We did: four blastocysts of good quality had made it to day five and were being frozen as we spoke. This would allow my body to have a month off all the drugs and hormones and have a normal period before (hopefully) getting pregnant. What a treat.

Phase Three: The Transfer

As weird as it sounds, my son was created almost a year to the day before he was born. By October 2019, our little embryos were safe in some sort of ice tray and I could have a lovely, restorative November menstrual cycle. Our initial plan was to go back in for the final procedure in December. If it worked – that big IF – it meant I would be about three weeks pregnant at Christmas.

At this news I went in on myself a little bit, fretting over the different scenarios, until my husband finally dragged out of me why I was worried.

'I know it sounds stupid, but if I'm a couple of weeks pregnant on Christmas Day, all the family will notice I'm not having fizz and guess that I'm up the duff. Then there'll be a big fuss but it'll be way too early to tell anyone as it could all be over by the New Year. I just don't think I'm ready to tell anyone yet.'

He smiled. 'Is that what's been bothering you?'

'A little bit.' I shrugged, aiming for aloof.

We chatted about it, and we realised that not much in this whole endeavour had been in our control. From the start we'd been at the behest of the next available appointment and the hospital's schedule. We'd even been slaves to my menstrual cycle and nature's timing for intercourse. I couldn't physically interfere in the internal process of getting the sperm to where it needed to be and naturally becoming pregnant. *When* to have the embryo transferred was one of the few things that was actually within our influence.

'Let's take a break,' he said.

So that's what we did. We had what would hopefully be our final Christmas, just the two of us, with friends and family. We ate, drank and were merry, and even travelled to Budapest in January as a final blowout before the ultimate hurdle in trying to conceive: the transfer. In my mind, the pregnancy was just a short hop, step and a jump between us and holding my baby for the perfect photo op, as a family of three, around our glittering tree.

I decided 2020 was going to be our year.

An infectious disease caused by the SARS-CoV-2 coronavirus on the other side of the world was starting to have other ideas.

My transfer was scheduled for the first week of February. What we didn't know was that just a few weeks later, all IVF treatments would be postponed due to Covid. We were incredibly lucky; a sliding doors moment, really. With my eyes on the prize, I faithfully jabbed myself and took the pills before I headed back to the clinic one more time for the big finale. Hopefully, we wouldn't need an encore.

My husband was allowed in the operating theatre this time and I begged him to make sure I didn't say anything stupid while I was off my tits on fentanyl. He made no promises. My body was technically five days pregnant. Hopefully, I'd created a nice little nest in there that the embryo would happily burrow into for the next nine months. Although it's ten really, isn't it? I don't know why we say nine months. It's forty weeks; my maths is abysmal but even I know forty divided by four equals ten. Anyway, I was prepped, dressed and ready to go. We had to wait around a while, so we made each other laugh inside our private curtained booth. He snapped pictures of me taking the piss out of those women who act heavily pregnant at three months. You know the ones, where they lower themselves into a chair backwards – with absolutely no bump – exaggeratingly grunting and moaning. I wouldn't find this so funny in about five weeks' time when I couldn't lift my head out of the toilet.

The protocol was to take an embryo out of the freezer, check it under the microscope and whip it across to me lying prone in theatre. It had to be quick. There was a clock on this. At this point the embryo would be one-tenth the size of a full stop and I'm ashamed to admit that for a long time, I thought some poor sod had to place it up into me by eye. I'm an idiot – there's cameras and all sorts. I needn't have fretted that someone needed to have the steadiest hand in the west. With a final nod from us, the embryologist went to get our first potential baby and said she'd be right back in five minutes.

But she wasn't back in five, ten or even twenty minutes. Eventually the blue curtain was drawn back by a nurse to reveal a very sombre-looking embryologist who suggested we should go into a side room. Ah, shit. It was The Sad Room – they were taking us into The Sad Room. I'd seen *Casualty*. We sat and faced her as she explained that 'unfortunately . . .' – never a good start from a medical professional – 'the first embryo didn't quite thaw how we would like.'

Okay . . . What the hell does that mean?

She explained that they hoped to observe the embryo collapse in on itself under the microscope during the thawing process and while it's not a total dud, it's not ideal.

Okay . . . What the hell does that mean?

She said they could either carry on with that embryo or thaw a second to see if it reacted better. She kept talking about the quality of the first being poor and I wondered if she was dissing my potential baby. What's a poor-quality baby anyway? Should I ask? We agreed to go for Door Number 2. Heading back to our cubicle to await the Great Second Thaw, we discussed what we would do if this one didn't work either. We had four to play with. Like bizarre chips at a high-stakes roulette table. Fifteen minutes later, the curtain was pulled back and the embryologist gestured to The Sad Room again. For fuck's sake. We sat facing her, once more, and she explained that 'unfortunately' – there's that word again – the same thing had happened with embryo number two. So, we could either proceed with thawing a third or put the two current defrosting ones in to give me a better chance.

Okay . . . What the hell does that mean?

My husband looked at me to suggest that it was entirely my

IVF

decision, but his eyes were screaming, 'Please don't pick the twin option.' I left him squirming for a little bit (because it was fun), but then said I thought we should try the third one. He released the breath he'd been holding, and I laughed, telling him there was still a chance this one wouldn't work either and we'd have to bung all three up there. I enjoyed watching the colour draining from his face. The embryologist continued to talk about the quality of the embryo and my brain was yelling at me to just ask.

'When you say quality, do you mean quality of child?'

She tried to hide her grin and remain professional.

'No, I'm sorry, I should have been clearer. When we're talking about quality, we're only talking about the viability of it becoming a pregnancy. You can have a low-quality embryo that continues to full term and produces a perfectly healthy baby.'

Ah, okay. Glad I asked. We decided on number three and went back to the bed and waited. This time when the curtain was ripped back, the embryologist was beaming.

'It collapsed beautifully.' Not a sentence you hear every day.

Numero Tres it was, then. I couldn't quite cope with the idea of giving birth to a litter, so we said goodbye to numbers one and two and it looked like we were going home with number three. Just like on *Blind Date*.

My bed was wheeled into the operating room and my husband held my hand as they showed us a tiny bubble on a big TV screen. That was our baby. The staff placed my feet in the stirrups, as it's one of those half beds where it runs out just after your bum. Then the nurses began whispering to each other and sharing concerned looks. Oh god, what now? I looked to my husband, and he tried to comfort me by saying everything would be fine. I looked back just as a nurse approached, discreetly bending down to my ear to whisper, 'You've left your knickers on.'

I laughed and, red-faced quickly removed my underwear while my husband stuffed them in his jeans pocket muttering what an idiot I was. I got back into position ready for the sedative to hit my system.

I woke up a while later to discover that I had talked a pile of shit *again*, and that we were now allowed to go home. Was I pregnant? What was I supposed to do now? Could I sit up like normal? Suddenly I was that annoying woman in early pregnancy who's forgotten how to sit. They gave me a bunch of leaflets and yet more drugs. One of the top FAQs was 'can the embryo fall out?' and I breathed a sigh of relief that I wasn't the only idiot to have wondered that, and it would save me an embarrassing Google search later.

I was handed a big paper bag. This was an exciting addition: pessaries. Yes, twice a day for the next twelve weeks, I would need to push a little soapy bullet up my arse. The romance of Vienna felt a lifetime ago. But it would support the lining of the womb, so I happily agreed to do it.

Alright, a couple did pop out, but by week two, I was a pessary pro.

Years later, I would discover these should have been inserted into the vagina – obviously. I don't know what to say in my defence.

I'm a literal and figurative arsehole.

2

A Pregnant Pause

(Or The World Goes to Hell in a Handbasket)

You're implored, as you leave the hospital, to wait two weeks before taking a pregnancy test, as they can not only give false positives but also false negatives. Naturally, I took a pregnancy test that same day. It was negative (of course). This was the '2ww' (Two-Week-Wait) on Mumsnet. Basically you need to become a Bletchley codebreaker to decipher the acronyms on that site. DD and DS denote Darling Daughter/Son. DH is Darling/Dear Husband, a phrase I swear to you, I will never use. There's the inevitable AIBU (Am I Being Unreasonable), usually the answer is a firm yes. There are perfectly reasonable contractions such as VBAC (Vaginal Birth After C-section), SALT (Speech and Language Therapist) or MW (Midwife). It goes from barely concealed, passive–aggressive HTH (Hope This Helps) and YABOS (You Are Being Overly Sensitive) to the totally bizarre, such as NAK (Nursing at Keyboard), EWCM (Egg White Cervical Mucus) and my favourite, JFGI (Just Fucking Google It).

I did – that's what led me to this hellhole.

The Two-Week Wait is like one of those comedy videos on YouTube that were a trend for a while. You set up a camera and carefully explain to a six-year-old that if they don't eat the delicious cupcake in front of them while you pop out for a few minutes, they can have two cupcakes on your return. Unsurprisingly, most of the time they can't resist and gobble it down. When the adult re-enters the room enquiring where the cake has gone, the child gives a shrug with big innocent eyes licking at the pink icing all around their chops. That was essentially me, every morning, post-embryo transfer. Running to the bathroom for my first wee of the day and holding the juicy cupcake of a fresh pregnancy test in my hands.

For every day of the first week, it was a negative. I was under no illusions that my husband wasn't fully aware of what I was doing, but even he could sympathise, what with how close we were and all. Nearly four years, or more precisely forty-six periods, of disappointment and defeat and there could be a tiny life inside me *right* now. I had to know. One morning, I prepared for another let-down but, wait a minute, was that a second line? It was so faint, I wondered if it was the sleep in my eyes. But my heart leapt – I couldn't believe it! Was I holding a positive pregnancy test? Was I pregnant? I didn't *feel* pregnant, but what the hell did I know? Each day I did another test, and each passing day that second line grew a little darker, a little more defined, until finally there was no denying it: I was holding in my hands a BFP (Big Fat Positive). I ran to our room, jumped on my husband in the bed, and beamed broadly as I held up the marvellous magic stick, the proof of our future happiness. The future, it seemed, smelt faintly of urine.

A PREGNANT PAUSE

★

In the first few weeks of my pregnancy, a terrible flood hit our town. Not a metaphor – an actual flood. Storm Dennis did a real number on Pontypridd and destroyed hundreds of homes and businesses. We live higher up, on a hill, away from the River Taff, but our old house along the riverbank was utterly ruined. It was a dark time for our whole community. My husband and I volunteered at the makeshift emergency centre, collecting and organising donations, shuttling things around, anything we could, really. Everything from cleaning products and non-perishable foods to, poignantly, newborn onesies were donated in droves. Some families lost everything. We morbidly joked that this flood was a biblical omen for my pregnancy.

The flood waters and damaged houses became more and more contaminated. My husband pleaded with me to stop delivering care packages to the affected areas. He would do it; could I please stay put in the community centre, where I was safe, and catalogue the donated items instead? Local people had rallied immediately and were being incredibly generous, so we essentially had a rudimentary supermarket with different departments: shoes, clothing, appliances, food and drink and even toys and books.

During this time, I was growing more and more nauseous, but instead of worrying about feeling crappy, I was elated. I was finally that pregnant protagonist in all those books and films I love so much. The comedy puking-in-a-bin-while-slowly-turning-green-as-someone-bores-you-with-their-fascinating-take-on-the-monarchy or not-able-to-hold-down-a-biscuit tropes were in full swing. I welcomed it all. It meant it was real and I was *so* excited.

The monarchy was a hot topic as the then Prince Charles

visited our hometown to regally survey the hammering it took. I was in the crowd above Prince's Café, a famous haunt in the Valleys as the art-deco tearooms, which have been going since 1948, were now flooded out. I was with my dad, who didn't know I was pregnant, and my husband, who was quietly trying to soothe the onslaught of my morning sickness. I vividly remember thinking how weird it was that I wanted to vomit all over the cobbled road of Market Street while everyone gawked for a glimpse of the future king. A stately visit from the sovereign was surely bad omen number two. This was fairytale stuff. Maybe I should request he lay his healing hand on my head to protect my pregnancy. A royal touch for the King's Evil. No, I wouldn't let any thoughts of pessimism enter the picture. I may have felt like death warmed up, but I also felt immensely lucky to feel so.

I continued to spend a fortune on, and take, pregnancy tests to reassure myself that it wasn't a mere figment of my imagination. I was being monitored by the clinic, and they tested my hCG (human chorionic gonadotropin) levels regularly to ensure the pregnancy was progressing nicely. Your hCG levels should sharply increase in the first eight to twelve weeks until they begin to level off. From week to week, they double, triple, even quadruple in number. From week five to week six the number rockets from around an average of 1,500 to 6,500, then 20,000 in week seven onwards to 80,000 in week eight.

*

At around six to seven weeks into my pregnancy, I had a blood test in Cardiff before travelling via Megabus to London for a voiceover. I was doing a few lines as some sort of supernatural creature in a new video game. Jobs had been few and far between lately, so it was either a tenner on the coach or the best part of a hundred pounds by train, and I couldn't really justify the latter with a baby on the way. Wandering around the streets of London with this little secret put a small smile on my lips and a skip in my step. I was doing it. I was a working actress in the Big Smoke with a baby on the way. I *was* having it all: climbing up through a precarious but artistic industry *and* starting a family with my other person on the planet. I couldn't wait.

At the fancy recording studios in Soho, I gave my name at the desk and took a seat, awaiting my turn. I heard someone holler, 'Kim!' I realised it must be someone I knew, as generally people I've just met in the business use my professional name, Kimberley. I looked up and saw an old friend, a smiling Maggie Service. In 2008 we had starred in *The Girl with a Pearl Earring* at the Haymarket Theatre in London. It had been a wonderful job with a great bunch of actors, including Adrian Dunbar as Vermeer and a young Jonathan Bailey, who would later go on to be the huge star of, well, everything: *Jurassic Park*, *Wicked*, *Bridgerton*. We had such a fun time doing that play. Creatively, it had been a bit challenging, to say the least, but as a cast, my goodness, did we laugh. So, to see Maggie again after all this time was a real treat. We chatted until she was called in first to record her voiceover. I said I'd see her afterwards for more of a catch-up, but as you'll find out, that catch-up wouldn't happen for a few more years.

As Maggie disappeared into the studio, my phone rang. It was the clinic. I knew I'd better take it as you can't possibly return their call through their complicated hospital switchboard, and it might have taken them a whole day to call back. Stealing a glance at the closed studio door and assuming they were just calling like every other time to confirm everything was on track or to maybe book in for another scan, I answered. The sober voice that greeted me didn't beat around the bush. After confirming my name and date of birth, they told me that they were sorry to inform me that my hCG levels had dropped 'significantly'.

'What does that mean?' I asked, scared as I could already guess the answer.

'Well, it's likely a sign that you're going to miscarry.'

Oh. I thought it had all been going too well. She pressed on, telling me that she would book me in for an early pregnancy scan first thing Monday morning to ensure the prognosis was correct and that no dangerous 'materials' were left behind. This is called RPOC, retained products of conception. Nice. She continued by saying that over the weekend, when the miscarriage would begin, I should head straight to A&E. Someone else was calling my name now, someone I didn't know as they were asking for Kimberley. Shit, the voiceover. I now had to pretend to be a fucking fairy. As quietly as possible, I quickly asked what questions I could think of on the spot, ended the call and headed into the booth.

Throughout the recording session I was on one side of the glass and the producers and engineers were on the other directing me via a speaker. I remember achieving the most incredible feat. When my emotions swelled up, I managed to cry only out of my right eye. I was facing the monitors in the tiny room, with only my left side visible to them. I still don't know how I pulled it off, and I can guarantee you I wouldn't be able to replicate it again. But it was unthinkable to be unprofessional and perhaps get a bad reputation as 'emotional' or 'unreliable'. This industry may be predicated on telling stories of the human condition, but it rarely allows room for flaws or circumstance in the production of it.

I got through it, stumbled out onto the cold London street and called my husband. I gently told him they thought I was losing our baby. He assured me it would be okay and told me to just head home. On the bus, I sank into the fuzzy seat, huddling to make myself as small as possible, and gazed out of the window at the passing orange lights along the M4. I usually read some trashy romance or watched a few episodes of something on my trips to and from London, but I just couldn't concentrate. We texted back and forth as I *never* talk on the phone on public transport. I never will. We each tried to console the other with the usual: 'at least I wasn't that far along', 'we'll try again', 'it's just one of those things'. We didn't believe any of it. The truth was that our hearts were beginning to break but that was okay – we were about to lose something unspeakably precious.

I was also shitting myself about the physicality of a miscarriage. What would happen? Would it hurt? Would I see anything? A tiny form in the blood? I googled 'Miscarriage, 6–7 weeks'. Take it from me, don't do that. I ventured back to Mumsnet, looking for an iota of hope, a kernel of proof that it didn't have to mean what they were telling me it did. I read thread after thread. I saw the same story again and again. Dropping hCG levels – especially a drop as steep as mine – meant it's over. Or it very soon would be. This was a Thursday night; we would have to wait until Monday morning for the scan. We were in for one of the worst weekends of our lives.

My husband and I were very gentle with each other over the next few days. There was none of the usual playful banter. We were just waiting for it to happen. I was scared, worried in some way that I would get the miscarriage wrong. Not do it properly, maybe, or even fail at it. I prayed my body would just know what to do. Because I sure as hell didn't.

We cwtched up and watched movies. Every time I went to the loo, I braced myself before I looked down. By Sunday evening, I started getting sharp pains. I called out for my husband, he raced to me and I tearfully explained, 'I think it's happening.'

'It's okay, Kimbo, everything's going to be okay.'

He only calls me Kimbo when I'm fragile.

No blood, or anything else for that matter, came, but I read that that wasn't unusual. The next morning, we trundled to the hospital, sad but ready to put this all behind us. We would take a break and maybe try another round of IVF somewhere down the road with our fourth and final frozen embryo. The future I'd imagined had dissipated in a puff of smoke and we sat in the grim, shabby waiting room. Holding hands, our fingers entwined, we waited and waited. I just wanted to go home and put my pyjamas on. Finally, my name was called – Kimberley – definitely not a friend, then. I got comfortable on the bed and the sonographer informed us that she'd be quiet for the next ten minutes or so while she scanned all the images, moving the vaginal probe around inside me. I was an old hand at this part now. Too sad to flinch, I looked up at the stained ceiling, occasionally at my husband's forlorn but supportive expression, all while we continued to hold hands. Just tell us already. The best-case scenario was that nature had taken its miserable course, and I wouldn't need any interventions.

A PREGNANT PAUSE

What felt like hours ticked by. The room was quiet, apart from the rustle of the hilariously useless modesty tissue-paper covering my lower half and the sonographer tapping away at her keyboard. She finally looked up and said, 'Okay . . .'

We both sat up. This was it. She started to turn the monitor around to face us and I thought to myself, 'What the hell is she doing? I don't want to look in there!' Would I see the remains of something? Or was she just proving it was empty, like a magician showing you the inside of his top hat before pulling out a white rabbit? It seemed like a particularly cruel trick when the illusionist already knew the little bunny had absconded. I kept my focus on my husband's face. I didn't want to look. I could always read his countenance like a book; his expression would be all I needed to know.

'That's your baby, guys.'

I glanced back. Is she taking the piss?

'See that little flicker, there?'

We both dumbly nodded. We could sort of see *something* moving. If we squinted.

'That's your baby's heartbeat. And it's strong and healthy . . .'

We were stunned. In the truest sense of the word. Speechless, which as you can probably tell, is a rarity for me. Hope began to bloom in my chest. She printed pictures and congratulated us. We staggered out, suppressing our giddiness. Was this real? I was supposed to go straight upstairs to the fertility clinic with the results so they could log it as a 'failed cycle', so up we went. We were met by a sympathetic-looking nurse, awaiting our arrival.

'It's all fine,' I blurted. 'The baby is fine. She said it's all healthy and fine.'

She looked shocked then sceptical. She looked to my husband;

he nodded, assuring her I hadn't gone mental and the baby was, indeed, fine. She was flabbergasted and popped off to tell some other member of staff. The paperwork suddenly changed, and we had to book in for yet more scans and monitoring while the sad 'failed attempt' form was put on ice. Presumably next to our remaining, now unneeded, fourth embryo. We left the hospital and, with a timely sprinkle of pathetic fallacy, the grey and dreary morning had transformed into a bright, sunny day. The magic was back; the rabbit was in there all the time. Tricky little leporine bastard.

*

In the next few weeks, not only did our lives change, but the entire world changed too. Boris Johnson addressed the nation – we were going into what they were calling a 'lockdown'. As Covid-19 hit with full force, pregnant women were placed on the vulnerable list. They didn't know the effects this unknown virus could have on the mother or foetus, so we were advised not to go near anyone. Fine by me. I continued to have severe morning sickness right up until eighteen weeks. Morning sickness, my arse; I was nauseous twenty-four/seven, a pallid grey colour and off most foods. I lay on the garden swing most days, as the rocking seemed to offset the unrelenting internal sway. Apart from the swing, there were only three things that seemed to help: ginger ale or ginger biscuits (honestly, I'd lick Ginger Spice if I thought it would lessen my queasiness); scratching the skin of a lemon and inhaling the scent deeply, which meant I was now the weirdo that carried a lemon in her pocket; and watching *The Vicar of Dibley*, sideways. Don't ask me why. I was also hit with pregnancy migraines and had to lie in a dark room for days at a time like a Victorian confinement. It was a very fun period.

A PREGNANT PAUSE

During lockdowns, everyday normal life was suspended for everyone. I couldn't see my dad, my in-laws, our nieces or nephews. My entire industry was virtually stood down, and I lived from day to day, pregnancy- and Covid-wise. We awaited the latest list of regulations, the most recent cans and can'ts, and saw more and more of my maternity rights go down the swanny. Midwife appointments were done via phone or masked up. You could go for one hour of exercise a day and almost the entire nation exhausted Netflix. Watching *Tiger King* at the same time as millions of strangers while growing a baby was almost a fever dream.

Every facet of our lives and culture was suspended or dismantled over the next six months. I had to pass my dad his birthday presents through the kitchen window; he couldn't blow out the candles on the Victoria sponge I'd proudly baked him, not if we all wanted to eat a slice, anyway. He wafted them out with his birthday card and it was one of the saddest things I'd ever seen. I was pregnant and queasy and just wanted a hug from my dad, but we would have been breaking the actual law. At one point we had a pathetic socially distanced family picnic. Legally everyone had to be six feet apart. My dad is about six foot so I had to imagine him lying on the floor, and I stayed about a dad away from everyone. In supermarkets, coffee shops, chemists, I was constantly envisaging being the length-of-my-dad apart from the person in front. Why not think of my husband? This was a barely veiled dig as he's 5 ft 11 and a half, as I liked to remind him regularly. So, a dad-away from everyone it was.

*

One day I woke up and the nausea was gone. The queasiness and the unyielding sickliness had vanished, and I bounced out of bed like a Disney fucking princess. I had a newfound joie de vivre. It was the summer, we were about to find out if we were having a son or a daughter and, apart from the plague dominating the globe, things were on the up.

I went on long walks with Bobbie (a girl), an insanely loyal yet barking mad mix of German shepherd, Labrador and Border Collie. We got her from a farm near Rumney on my 'Birthday Boxing Day' in 2016, a term which my husband insists every year 'doesn't exist'. But everyone should have the day after their birthday be a time of left-over cake, playing around with presents and regret. She was the product of the two working farm dogs having relations and, as badly as I've trained her, I love her unconditionally. She's my shadow – she's been by my side since the day we went into the stables and the farmer said in a very Valleys accent, 'She'll be a lovely fawn bitch.' My ten-year-old (at the time) nephew and I giggled and I knew she was the one. She's dark blonde with big brown eyes, a bit like me, so my husband lovingly dubbed us the Fawn Bitches. She's the only one I want around me when the world gets a little too big sometimes. We named her after Bob, the canine protagonist in Agatha Christie's *Dumb Witness*, the infamous girl Bob in *Blackadder*, and the fact that if my husband had to yell her name across a park, he wouldn't – (and I quote) 'look like a knobhead'. We already had cats called Aggie and Hercule, he vetoed Missy after Jane Marple and so Bobbie it was.

On these lush, verdant walks, I listened to the same twenty songs. I like the familiar (see: TTC Romance Mix). A blend of everything from 'Alone Again (Naturally)' to 'Harper Valley P.T.A.', 'Gyp the Cat' to Tom Odell's 'Half As Good As You'. I could use this as my birthing playlist, I mused. (Top mental health tip: if you're feeling down, listen to 'Answering Machine' by Rupert Holmes – you know, the 'Piña Colada Song' guy. You're welcome.) My bump was growing and expanding and the more pregnant I looked, the greater I felt. I was flooded with superwoman hormones; the famed 'glow' was here. I'm not kidding, I looked fucking radiant. We prepared the nursery, washed all the tiny baby clothes, I read everything I could get my hands on about babies and birthing and parenting and raising a healthy, well-adjusted child. I had this in the bag.

Due to Covid, I had to attend every scan and antenatal appointment alone, which, while a little daunting, I didn't have any other pregnancy experience to compare it to. I headed into Llwynypia Hospital (CHLOYN-uh-peer), which all of Cwm Taf Morgannwg Healthboard's maternity had been diverted to. Half of the hospital was closed down due to Covid, with eerily dark corridors and silent, unused equipment. In the dimness, pregnant women waddled around trying to find the right room for a scan or consultation; it was like What to Expect When You're Expecting: Zombie Apocalypse.

The twenty-week scan, the fun one where you can find out the sex of the baby was, rather depressingly, called the Anomaly Scan. I've read that they measure the baby's bones and assess other developmental markers and look for possible 'structural defects'. Not something I wanted to be on my own for, but head held high, I strolled in all by myself, my husband's pep talk of 'don't take any shit' steeling my spine. He really is a man of few words. But I wasn't nauseous anymore, everything was progressing well and I was going to find out if I was having a little girl or boy. The sun was shining and there was a definite spring back in my step.

The waiting room was filled with bumps of various sizes

and as I took my seat, a tearful woman was escorted out of one of the scan rooms, having obviously just heard the worst news imaginable. That made me pause and I remembered that hospitals are a place of life *and* death. My name was called ten minutes later but my mind was still with that poor grieving mother. Looking at the ominous clinical door ahead of me, I swallowed. My turn.

I was nervous but I must confess, before arriving that day, the only numbers I'd been interested in were the cranial measurements, specifically the head circumference. How do I put this delicately? My husband and all the males in his family have massive heads and I wanted to be prepared for vaginal obliteration. Now, my sole focus was on hearing a heartbeat. Within a few minutes, thankfully, the glorious drone began to fill the room.

In amongst all the jargon the sonographer was calling out over his shoulder for the nurse to jot down, I caught that the HC was 16cms. Phew! That sounded normal. I'm not very good with measurements – distance, length, width, time – so my only barometer was the 30cm white plastic ruler we used in school (see also: measuring length in 'dads'). It was about half that, then. Okay. Not ideal but it seemed pushable.

The guy wielding the transducer was now pushing it firmly against my bursting belly – you're supposed to drink copious glasses of water beforehand and not pee, to create what radiographers playfully call an 'acoustic window'. Not only does it sound like a shit band at your local pub, it allows the fluid to push the intestines out of the way and for sound waves to travel, revealing a clearer image of the pelvic organs like the uterus and ovaries. But with a growing baby already playing keepy-uppy with your bladder, asking a pregnant woman to hold her pee is almost a form of torture. The sonographer was hidden behind a surgical mask and a full-face visor. Belt and braces. It was pretty hard to make out what he was saying but I *thought* he was asking if I wanted to know the sex. I gleefully told the medical team around me that I'd brought in a plain sheet of paper with an envelope, and would they mind writing down BOY or GIRL and sealing it so my husband and I could find out together later that evening. We'd have a celebratory dinner and try to make as much of an occasion of it as we could under the new decrees we were living under. A very mumbled 'that's against policy, sorry' was followed up by an almost bored 'do you still want to know?' Well, at least I heard that. Did I? I hadn't anticipated my request being so outlandish it would be met with such a blunt rebuff, especially considering the exceptional circumstances we found ourselves in, with all partners banned from attending scans.

He was looking at me impatiently. He wanted to move on. Shit, shit, shit, what should I say? I knew I didn't have any further scans scheduled, so the next time we could find out would be at the birth. Well, fuck that noise. This pregnancy had had enough surprise elements already. I nodded and said, 'Yes, please.' He looked back at the monitor and said:

'It's a bmmmmmmhh.'

Yep, I did not hear that. I pretended I had and smiled like I was delighted. I lay back and gave myself a stern mental talking to. Now was not the time to be polite and smile and blindly nod along. You *need* to know this piece of information. I imagined my husband, waiting in the car park, insisting I go back in and ask again, so with that mortifying idea bubbling away, I exclaimed, 'Sorry, I didn't hear you! Did you say "boy"?'

He nodded and, although his voice was still muffled, I heard a clearer, 'It's a boy!'

Whoa. We were having a little boy. I was going to have a son. I would be the mother of a son. Awesome, in the truest sense of the word.

It was a strange feeling having a definitive answer. For five months now we'd been saying he or she, thinking of girls' names as well as boys', imagining our potential future raising a son or a daughter. I had Schrodinger's baby inside me. Everything was possible. I had seen two paths ahead of me, and with one quick sentence, the entire girl/daughter path dissolved into wisps of nothingness. I had to walk the long and winding path to Boy Town – which, now I write it, sounds like a male strip club or cheesy nineties band. It was even stranger to have this knowledge all to myself for the next thirty minutes, while I swung by the consultant. Since the fun had been taken out of it for me, I decided to do a gender reveal of my own for my husband. It would involve an air rifle, a black balloon filled with blue confetti and, to be fair, absolutely impeccable aim. Even putting the unused pink confetti in the bin would feel weirdly final.

Leaving the hospital, I saw all the other dads hanging nervously around their parked cars, and it was then I noticed the woman who had left earlier. I walked by, trying not to intrude on their moment as her partner consoled her. She'd had to find out something devastating, all alone. Not only that but she'd then had to come out here and regurgitate it to, who I assumed was, the father. Guilt began to mushroom in my chest. Our baby was okay, theirs clearly wasn't. But us women were receiving momentous news, both joyful and tragic, and we were all doing it on our own. These new rules were beginning to make less and less sense to me.

I filmed the much-feted gender reveal and sent it to the family WhatsApp. As the blue scraps of paper flittered to the patio, I proclaimed, 'You're having a son!' to which my husband eloquently replied, 'Chuffed!', lowering the gun to his side with a wry smile on his face. A man of few words, indeed.

*

My third trimester arrived before I knew it, the slow drag of those first months entirely forgotten as we advanced steadily towards zero hour. I found myself writing to my MP, Alex Davies-Jones; I'd met her once or twice before and felt comfortable getting in touch about the worrying state of maternity care; my rights (or lack of) had left me feeling that I would have more say giving birth in a pub. At least then I could have people with me. My husband would be by my side. I wouldn't need a stranger's fingers shoved into my vagina to discover whether I'm the 5cm dilated required to allow my husband to legally join me at my bedside to give me some support. He also wouldn't be thrown out an hour after the birth. I thought about emailing Wetherspoons to see if we could come to some sort of an arrangement.

9 September 2020

Hi Alex,

I'm currently 33 weeks pregnant with our first baby
(after a lengthy IVF process) and my pregnancy has
pretty much run alongside lockdown. I wonder if you
have any plans to look into the lifting of restrictions on
antenatal/maternity care? I've attended every

appointment and scan alone and I will have to be on
my own for labour until I'm 5cm dilated. Only then
can my husband join me and then only stay for one
hour after the birth . . . It feels strange that we can go
to the pub, to restaurants, be on planes in close quarters
but birth partners/fathers can't provide emotional
support for pregnant women (especially those with
mental health issues) at such a uniquely vulnerable time.

They have now lifted the partner ban on the 12- and
20-week scans but other growth or anomaly scans still
have the restrictions in place. I just attended an
additional 32-week scan alone while in the waiting
room with women attending their 12/20 week scans
with their partners. It seems especially strange as if you
need extra monitoring, there's the chance something
may be wrong and having someone there to support or
advocate for you is even more crucial.

I appreciate your time and look forward to hearing
your views.

Kimberley Nixon
(Pontypridd resident)

Alex replied with a swift and compassionate response as she
thought 'there is a real case for partners to be able to attend',
but due to the devolvement of health in Wales to the Senedd
– as our Member of Parliament in Westminster – she was a
'tad limited'. But she insisted she had 'repeatedly' raised this

issue and promised to ask again in a meeting she was due to have with Cwm Taf Morgannwg Health Board. The ongoing message from them was that there was a danger to patients and staff but they were reviewing it.

9 September 2020

Hi Alex,

Thanks for getting back to me.

I completely understand the stance in relation to visitors or non-essential companions, but with the father of the baby, it doesn't seem right to keep them away from a) their newborn baby or b) their wife when she is going through the most life-changing and scariest of experiences, especially first-time mums.

The regulations in England are different, allowing two birth partners and visitors for an hour a day. With PPE and testing (the mums get tested before going in, why not the dads?), it would allow everyone to have peace of mind that it's a safe environment.

Scans, tests, induction, latent stage of labour (pre 5cms) are all being done by women on their own. There is also an issue around women who decline vaginal exams (due to sexual assault, risk of infection or a host of other reasons) who are feeling forced into them in order to check they're over the 4cm mark so that their partner can finally join them. I hate to think of the fallout from all of this in relation to post-natal depression and mental health. I had a CTG today due to a change in foetal movements (everything was absolutely fine!) but I did think of those women who have to go out to the hospital car park and inform their partner that something is wrong or worst-case scenario, there's no heartbeat.

At the moment, when you're in labour, you're dropped off at the hospital entrance and then have to make/waddle your way through stairwells and endless corridors alone (with all your bags!) to make it to the maternity ward. Then if you have to stay in post-delivery, you're all alone with a newborn for days on end. There are some really frightened pregnant women in Cwm Taf right now.

I really appreciate you meeting with the Health Board and hope that these exceptions to the rule will come into play and allow women to feel supported and empowered through birth, not afraid and alone.

Hoping you and your family are safe and well, and thanks again for taking this on when you must be snowed under with a plethora of COVID-related issues.

Kim x

Again, I could not fault my MP's rapid and sincere reply. She largely agreed with all my points and assured me that they were 'constantly reviewing the situation'. Alex informed me that the concern lay in the amount of cleaning time between scans, which would increase if partners were allowed in, thus waiting lists would rise. She offered to put me in touch with Mick Antoniw AM (our Assembly Member for the Senedd) as he could raise points directly within the Welsh government. She promised to stay in touch and wished me well in my continuing pregnancy.

10 September 2020

Hi Alex,

Thanks for keeping me posted. This is very disappointing indeed and I'm not sure it makes all that much sense – 12- and 20-week scans are now allowing partners. Why not for people who need extra scans at 32 weeks? Also, it seems to me that if a room needs cleaning between appointments, it makes no difference if there were three people in there compared with two?! I'm still not quite seeing the logic in allowing partners in for the second half of labour but not from when the woman is admitted. There are no tests in place at present. So if the father of the baby has Covid-19, they're coming in anyway from 4cms onward. Why not test and use PPE to make it safer all round and a better experience for the woman during the whole of her labour?

I completely understand not allowing endless visitors on maternity wards but one visitor for one hour a day in PPE seems completely reasonable and I'm sure allows speedier recoveries for the mums and bonding time for the dads.

The issue of vaginal examinations is also placing vulnerable women in a catch-22 position. You can't have your partner with you for an intimate – and for some women, psychologically difficult – examination, but without one, you're kept from your partner for longer.

I so appreciate you raising this issue with the Health Board and for looping me in. It's just disheartening that women seem to be at the bottom of the pile. Some women joke that they'd be better off giving birth in a pub as they'd have more rights. It feels like giving birth should be a special exception to the rules and that with strict measures around testing and PPE in place, this could be easily achievable. I can't imagine being in labour and being dropped at the hospital door with my bags and spending the next, however many, hours or days alone without the person I trust most in the world there to support me and advocate on my behalf.

I hope things will continue to be monitored and updated and that pregnant women in Wales are soon given back some much-needed rights.

Thanks again for the info,
Kim x

PS I'm happy for you to forward on these emails to Mick Antoniw AM.

A PREGNANT PAUSE

Within a day, she replied that she would, indeed, forward my emails to Mick Antoniw's office and sent 'dymuniadau gorau' (best wishes). My next communication was from my AM's case manager, who forwarded me the response they'd received from the Chair of the Health Board, Dr Marcus Longley.

Long email short, they had no plans to change the rules but conceded 'the points which your constituent makes about the importance also of attending later scans, and being present throughout birth, are well made'. However, the risk to staff, patients and the partners was 'still too great'.

In Wales during this time, as I've said, healthcare is devolved to the Welsh government; I could visit the pub or a restaurant with five friends or family members, but in order for my husband to gain entry to the hospital to hold my hand during the most vulnerable and potentially dangerous experience of my life, five is also the exact number of centimetres my cervix would need to be stretched to. My cousin in England (who was also named Kimberley, but without the second E – long story!), was pregnant at the same time as me with her third child, and she was allowed to have two birth partners and a visitor while on the maternity ward but this was at the hospital's discretion, so again not across the board. It all seemed so chaotic and senseless.

My due date was in a month or so and regulations were changing week by week. I really wanted to know where I stood. My hospital bags were packed, everything labelled inside so it would be easier for hospital staff to retrieve things from my suitcase without a birthing partner there to help. Despite this ongoing to-ing and fro-ing, I was getting even more excited to meet my baby, to finally have him in my arms where he belonged.

The final weeks passed in a blur. We had a babymoon/birthday stay over in a hotel twenty minutes from our house as we weren't allowed to leave the county. I had a splendid bubble bath in the clawfoot tub and tried pigeon in the fancy restaurant (it was nothing to write home about). And then, suddenly, it was the eve of the birth. I was having a planned C-section the next day. The reason was primarily because of potential placenta previa (where the placenta is essentially in front of the baby, blocking the exit). I also didn't think I would physically be able to handle the vaginismus they suspected I had, meaning sweeps and fingers for dilation checks were a scary prospect. If they couldn't say how far along in labour I was, I would be on my own as birth partners could only be present from 5cm dilated (sorry to keep labouring the point, pun intended). Add to that a complete lack of consistency in Covid regulations and a diagnosis of tokophobia (fear of physically giving birth – as a little girl of eight or nine, I'd spend nights lying awake worrying about giving birth one day in the far-off future), they had agreed that an elected Caesarean would be best. My husband could be there with me throughout and up to an hour after the birth. I'd heard horror stories of local women being induced and left on their own in hospital for three days in early labour. We ordered a curry and watched *Iron Man 2*. I imagined Mary and Joseph having a similar sort of evening the night before the big day.

I got into bed and looked at the crib next to me, ready and waiting with fresh sheets and a tiny sleeping bag. Tomorrow I would be a mother, and I just couldn't wait. After wedging the enormous pregnancy pillow under my bump, I turned off the light, smiling to myself. But then my eyes sprang open in the darkness. Could I still listen to my Agatha Christie audiobooks every night with a baby here? With that small niggle burrowing in my brain, I drifted off to sleep.

3

The Golden Hour

(or The Loneliest Poo of Your Life)

The Golden Hour is the one to two hours following birth when you can indulge in precious skin-to-skin time with your baby. This promotes the feel-good hormone, oxytocin. This cherished period should also help you regulate after the birth and encourage breast-feeding and bonding to begin. Sometimes called Kangaroo Care, Dads are encouraged to go skin-to-skin with the baby too, held upright on their bare chest. All very delicious-sounding and nurturing. Nourishment for the soul.

Unfortunately for me, shortly after giving birth to my son, something deep inside me glitched so completely and so entirely, it was like flipping a switch. One minute my son was being held up by the doctor in a Simba-esque pose for everyone to bask in his awe – my long-awaited baby boy, handed to me for the first hold – the next minute I was slurring, 'Take the baby, take the baby, take the b . . .' and I was gone.

I was bleeding out.

The room became a chaotic scramble, with people trying to figure out where the bleed was coming from and what drugs

I'd been given (someone had been a bit lax on keeping a tight record of that), and my husband standing still in the middle of all of it, clutching this tiny bundle I'd all but thrown at him.

If I were to shoot this scene, this singular moment, the camera would do a 180-degree flip so the whole world jolted upside down. The glorious technicolour of bright surgical lights, blue scrubs and a crimson-covered baby would drain itself of all life and colour. The world became an indistinguishable mass of grey, not the golden hues I was promised.

When I came round, I was told I'd lost too much blood. I needed two transfusions and because of that, as a treat, the Welsh government would let my husband stay with me for a little longer, rather than him swiftly being kicked out due to Covid regulations. So, there I was, in a private room next to the operating theatre, blood going in and milk coming out. My wee was being collected in a lovely little bag hanging off the bed and a midwife was clamping my son to my boob. Golden Hour, my arse.

The baby attached himself to my nipple. 'Holy shit, what is this?' I thought, as pain zipped through me. It hurt. Not in a 'there's a slight discomfort to start but it'll soon fade and you'll be fine' way. I mean, it *really fucking hurt*. It was like a wooden, gummy vice had been clamped down on my tit. This wasn't the most natural thing in the world – it was torture. But I didn't say anything. I just gazed down at his pudgy, perfect little face and thought, 'It's okay, he's here and it'll get better.'

But the world around me wasn't sitting right. It was off by a degree or two and, like in *The Truman Show*, I was the only one who seemed to notice. Either that or everyone else was pretending, but why would they be doing that to me? The nurse escorted my husband to do the first nappy change and it was a cute moment. I was snapping away on my phone from across the room and trying not to giggle because I knew the first poo – the meconium – would be black and sticky. I knew he would be internally gagging and thinking it was gross but trying to keep a straight face in front of the staff. By the way, in the first week of a baby's life, they'll try to flummox you with what should be happening poo-wise to ensure the baby is healthy. Let me save you a hundred quid on an antenatal class and tell you the general rule of thumb: Marmite to pesto to korma. However, as this adorable scene was playing out on one side of the room, I was starting to feel like a glass wall was descending, cutting me off from the people right in front of me. Although everyone could see me, they were now somehow out of my reach.

Then all hell broke loose.

The cute, gurgly sound our new baby had been making, dismissed by the midwives thus far, suddenly piqued the attention of the doctor who had just entered. Before we knew what was happening, a paediatric team swooped into the room and began discussing our son with an urgency to their voices. The main doctor turned to us and said – through a surgical mask and a visor – 'something's wrong' . . . 'breathing difficulties' . . . 'possible sepsis' . . . Wait, did he just say sepsis? It was so hard to tell through the actual and metaphorical barriers that divided us.

The transparent cot containing my tiny, ever-so-vulnerable baby was wheeled out of the room. My husband was given an almost impossible choice. Like a grotesque game show, he was told that the baby was going to the SCBU – where? – and his wife couldn't be moved due to the ongoing blood transfusions, so who did he want to stay with? The catch? Whoever he chose would be the only one he could see from now on. Due to Covid, he wouldn't be allowed to travel between the two of us, so he would have to stay either with his newborn son or the great love of his life (my words, not his).

The paediatric team were leaving with our baby, so he had to decide – quickly. I pushed him towards the door, reassuring him I would be fine and insisting he remained with the baby no matter what and to text me constant updates. He stumbled out after them, the door closing with a finality to his decision. I was suddenly all alone, in a sterile, unfeeling room, my guts basically hanging out and a stranger's blood being pumped into me with the worrying suspicion that that was the last time I would ever see my little boy alive.

Shit, that escalated fast.

I spent the next hour or so slowly and entirely collapsing in on myself, like that third embryo that was now a defenceless little baby, lost to me, somewhere in this 1970s brutalist building. There was an unnerving Soviet feeling to the place both architecturally and in atmosphere. Nurses came and went as they checked on me; I think one stayed chatting to me for a while. I don't know. I wasn't really there. I was texted updates of my son's progress. I kept begging my husband to send me pictures and I couldn't understand his reluctance unless . . . well, you couldn't really WhatsApp a photo of a dead baby to a woman who'd just given birth to it, I guess. That would be insensitive. He was protecting me; he didn't know how to tell me. That's what it was, I painfully concluded.

The door kept opening, and each time I braced myself for

the sympathetic face of a stranger to break the news, in heavily clinical terms, that my baby hadn't made it. I called my husband over and over. He wasn't picking up. Yep, of course he couldn't answer – there were probably dead baby forms to fill out and he'd want to tell me face to face. My thoughts were getting darker; I was spiralling. Suddenly he was calling me back, telling me everything was fine, but I didn't believe it. He was probably just trying to keep me calm. Yet another nurse came into the room. Was this it? No, she was just checking my chart. I figured they must have wanted to wait until I wasn't alone to tell me. I was so incredibly scared and beyond sad. And the lingering thought was that I couldn't quite remember my baby's face.

My husband told me that he didn't want to send a picture because he thought it would worry me. Well, yes, a picture of my precious lifeless baby probably would have worried me. Good call. He told me that our baby had a tube up his nose and that it 'looked worse than it is'. What an odd way of putting it. Then he told me he'd send a photo through now. I still couldn't picture his face; his tiny, scrunched-up old man-like face. Identical to Winston Churchill. Most babies look like Winston Churchill when they're born, don't they? Now I was just thinking of Churchill's face on a baby's body, and I didn't want to remember my son that way. I shook away the image and pulled up pictures that were taken hours ago. Oh yes, that was his face. I kept staring at it. Kept remembering. I closed my eyes. I couldn't do this. I wouldn't survive this. We wouldn't even be able to give him a proper funeral. Only fifteen people were allowed to attend under current restrictions. He never even got to meet fifteen people.

Ping!

I looked down at the phone clutched in my hand. My husband had sent me a message: a picture of a baby. Not just a baby. *My* baby. It felt weird. I didn't feel like a mother yet. When would that kick in? Would it ever kick in if I was only a mum for such a short time? 'How is Mum?' I kept getting asked that. All the staff were suddenly calling me 'Mum'. I was Kim about four hours ago. Now, I was simply 'Mum' and he was 'baby'. What the fuck happens to the definite article when you enter a medical setting? 'How is Mum?' I didn't know. Not very good, I didn't think. I was clearly not a good mum; I'd already ruined this whole thing. I must have done something wrong.

The cherubic little face in the picture had his eyes closed. That made sense. He had some intrusive tubing shoved up his nose. It didn't seem to be bothering him. That made sense, too. I just stared. We'd been so close; we nearly had our little family, and it felt cruel to have it taken away now. There was writing beneath the picture but I couldn't focus enough to read it. Another nurse came in. I waited. She didn't deliver the news either. Why was no one telling me? I refocused. The message read that he was okay. They were just monitoring him. He was 'grunting'. It's common with C-section babies apparently. Lingering lung fluid. He was fine. It would pass. He was perfect.

That couldn't be right.

He was fine. My baby was not dead. My baby was fine. I said it over and over and over again in my head. Trying it on for size. Trying to make my body believe it. He was going to be fine. Thank God. But where was the whoosh of relief? Where was the gargantuan weight off my shoulders? It wasn't lifting. Why wasn't it lifting?! I kept getting messages. Congratulatory ones from friends and family. Reassuring ones from my husband. But still, something was off. And again, no one could see it but me.

After the second transfusion was finally complete, I was allowed to go to the baby unit. My husband and I were like ships in the night. For me to be able to enter and see the baby, he had to pass by me and leave. He reassured me again. Told me he was perfect. Told me he loved me, he was so proud of me, and he'd see me tomorrow. We didn't know, yet, that that wasn't true.

And then I was alone again. It was one thirty in the morning. Our son was the only baby in the ward. The lights were dimmed, the voices of the nurses hushed as they chatted around their workstation, and I could hear his steady little heartbeat in the form of a comforting beep. But I wasn't comforted. I wasn't relieved. I didn't understand why I didn't feel better now that I could see with my own two eyes that he was, indeed, fine. I was tense from the roots of my hair to the tips of my scrunched-up toes. I didn't think I'd released a breath properly in hours.

Then I realised something. He was lying on his front. That was a big no-no. All the books said that – I'm a nerd and had done my homework. Even those horribly awkward Zoom NCT sessions said it. Feet to foot, so the baby's feet should be touching the foot of the cot and they should always, *always* be placed on their back. But he was on his front.

Panic started to rise; I was frozen. What should I do? I'd had abdominal surgery about nine hours ago. I was on my feet, but barely. In the end, a nurse floated over to check his vitals and I blurted it out. 'He's on his front!'

She looked back at me. I continued, trying to conceal my alarm. 'I thought they had to be on their backs?' I felt like I was silently screaming 'COT DEATH! COT DEATH!' at her. She just smiled warmly and explained that this was a special cot with a sensor mat. It would help with his breathing to be on his front, and he was constantly being monitored by staff and the machines – unlike at home – where I should indeed put him on his back.

Cot death. I knew it wasn't called that anymore, was it? It was a name, a boy's name . . . SIDS. That was it. What did that stand for, again? I knew D was for Death. What was the S and the I? Sleeping Induced Death? No, that didn't sound right. I tuned back in to realise the SCBU nurse had been talking to me the entire time. I looked around and my eyes landed on a horribly wipeable plastic armchair. Why wasn't there a bed for me? I wanted to stay here, next to him, to make sure he stayed alive. What was that? She was telling me that I needed to go back to the ward and sleep. It was 2am – I could see him in the morning. Could I sleep in the chair? No? Okay. I took more photos so I could remember his face this time, then slowly shuffled across the corridor into Ward 21.

It was deathly quiet apart from scattered beeps and whispers. I was led to a darkened room. The patients and new babies were all fast asleep. There were six beds in the room, three on each side facing each other. The middle beds were empty, due to Covid. The three other corners were occupied. I was directed towards the bed in the far-right corner. The nurse set my suitcase down and left. It was eerily quiet. I struggled onto the bed. I was in quite a lot of pain. I had a catheter in. I was exhausted but wired. I slowly reclined and for the next five hours, lay prone on top of the covers, staring at the ceiling. Almost catatonic. Every so often the gurgling sounds and hungry cries of the newborns pulled my attention back to the room but mainly I just waited. Waited for someone to come in and tell me he didn't make it. What should I say when they tell me? Would they let my husband back in to give me a hug? Would I have to hold him? Did I want to hold a dead baby? What if I didn't like holding him? What if I couldn't bring myself to give him back? I wondered what the law was on how long you could hold your deceased newborn before they were seized by the authorities. How many minutes between being a mother with parental rights to becoming an obstruction to hospital policy?

My descent into a terrifying vortex was gaining momentum when suddenly the hideous overhead fluorescent lighting groaned to life and staff began to bustle in. Was it not nighttime anymore? A lady came over to me with a notebook. I stared at her.

She smiled widely. 'Any tea for Mum?'

What the hell was she talking about? Who was Mum? Shit. That was me. She meant me. I wasn't a mum. I didn't even have my baby with me. He was all alone somewhere else. I don't really drink tea. I always have coffee in the morning. I said 'yes, please' to the tea.

I looked around at my fellow inmates. I felt locked in there – that's really what it felt like. We couldn't freely move around due to Covid, and everything was so clinical and institutionalised. One of my biggest fears has always been being sent to prison or a mental health facility for a crime I didn't commit. I hate those films – *Shawshank*, *Double Jeopardy*, *The Fugitive*.

I've never seen *The Green Mile*, I imagine I would hate it for this very reason.

It felt like a waking nightmare. My darkest fears made flesh, albeit a decaying one. My much-longed-for baby taken away from me and locked in a suffocating medical environment. Was this what hell was like? I struggled to sit up. I thought she was asking me about breakfast. Toast? Yeah, sure. She moved on to the next 'Mum' and asked about tea and toast, where she was greeted by a 'No, ta, got these', pulling out a pint-size can of Monster and a grab bag of beef Hula Hoops.

A nurse approached. A little paper cup with two pink pills was stretched out to me.

'Here's your Ibuprofen, love.'

Something was trying to penetrate the fog. I was remembering something. I'm sure I'd heard . . . oh, oh yeah.

'Can I have them now?' I frowned.

'Why wouldn't you be able to have them?'

'Because I had two blood transfusions last night.'

'Oh, did you? Hang on, let me check.'

I looked around at the other women. Babies next to them in uniform transparent, plastic cots. I felt so out of place.

She was back with a chart. 'You're right, you can't have them.'

She was leaving. Quick. Ask!

'Can I see my baby?'

'Where is it?' she enquired.

'Sk-boo?' Was I saying that right? SCBU is the Special Care Baby Unit. It's such a vague yet scary title.

'Oh right, well, you can go over after rounds.'

Pale tea and soggy toast landed on the vinyl-covered wheelie table set across the end of my bed. Right, breakfast. Come on.

Go through the motions. Be allowed out. I tasted nothing. I kept sipping my huge water bottle filled with blackcurrant squash — I hate water, it's so bland — as I read online that after birth, but particularly a C-section, the faster you can show you can pass urine and move your bowels, the quicker you'll get home. I chugged it.

I felt so strange. Like I was in a glass box. Nothing was quite landing with me. The surgeon who performed my Caesarean came by to do my post-op check-up.

'I hear you're an actress?' She grinned.

I smiled numbly in acknowledgement. She reminded me of Kate Burton (daughter of Richard) in Grey's Anatomy. But why are we talking about actresses again?

'Well, I've given you a very neat scar, so I hope you'll be happy with it?'

What? What was she talking about? Where the hell was my baby? I didn't give a shit about how pretty my scar would be or whether it would sit trimly beneath my bikini bottoms. Who gave a fuck? Mojitos and sarongs felt a world away right now. It was so hot in there. But not the soft, salty heat of a beach with the ocean lapping the shore. This heat was oppressive. I needed to get out of there. I asked again if I could go to see my baby. Someone would be around to let me know soon. I asked how he's doing. They weren't sure, they'd have to check. I looked at them blankly. Can you check please? Finally, a different nurse sidled up and told me he was fine. What did 'fine' mean? I say 'fine' a lot when I'm anything but . . . Was it one of those 'fines'?

I wanted to go and see him but apparently there were no wheelchairs available. Okay, I'd walk. I waited for someone to help me as I struggled, since I couldn't engage my abs to sit up. Nurses chatted over by the desk, seemingly not noticing that I was floundering about like an injured sea otter, trying to get out of bed. Eventually, I managed to put on my pink fluffy dressing gown and grabbed the full bag of piss with its direct line to my urethra and stuffed it into my pink fluffy pocket. My dressing gown looked too vibrant and out-of-place against this cold, unfamiliar background. It took me much longer than my normally spry walking pace to cross the short distance and make my way through the security buzzer outside the SCBU. I was still waiting for the other shoe to drop – for someone to bar my way because it would be too harrowing for me to see him, but everyone seemed calm and distracted by their own tasks.

I was allowed through and, as I rounded the corner, I saw him. So small, the steady beep telling my brain something my heart was too frightened to believe. I looked at him, at his tiny face. Did I love him? I thought so. I wanted to protect him, but I couldn't tell if I loved him more than anything else in the world yet. The breastfeeding nurse came in, an older lady with grey hair and a no-nonsense yet kind demeanour. Did I want to feed him? Shit. Breastfeeding. Yes, this was it. I'd breastfeed him and it would cement our bond and confirm to me that he was alive and well and we could go home and start our new lives together. I vaguely remembered some lovely, young trainee midwife massaging my boob and collecting the colostrum into little syringes to take over to the baby the night before, while I was hooked up to the transfusions. He'd got some golden goodness and now my milk would come in and I could start being a mother.

Settling into that horrid pastel-blue plastic armchair, a cushion was placed on my lap and my baby into my arms. Okay, this was it – we'd done it: IVF had worked, the pregnancy was done, the birth was over, and we'd survived the night – everything would be fine now. But why didn't I believe that? He was positioned to latch onto me. Somewhere in the back of my blurry mind 'nose to nipple' made me laugh. He started to feed and it was excruciating. We'd find out a few weeks later that he was tongue-tied and not latching 'perfectly' like I had been assured repeatedly. It was a strange sensation; milk being sucked out of you. There was an internal tickle in the centre of my boob I couldn't quite scratch, and my poor nipples became raw.

I was left to feed him, trying to enjoy it. I took a selfie to send to my husband to let him know we were both okay. He was coming in. He couldn't visit me on the ward but I promised him I was fine and that he should come in to see the baby. Once he arrived, I'd have to leave. Only one visitor at a time. Covid.

Looking down at the face of the little boy I'd created, with the help of my husband and some unknown lab technician, it came to me. I remember now. It was 'sudden' and 'instant'. Sudden Infant Death Syndrome. My belly filled with a deep, engulfing dread.

★

Back in my bed, breastfeeding continued to be agonising. A sweet trainee midwife helped me to express, so at least he was getting everything he needed from me via a small syringe. But the seed had been planted that I was a failure. I don't know if you've ever been milked by another human being, but it's as bizarre and undignified as it sounds. My breasts were tender to the touch, sore and swollen. My nipples, God bless them, grew redder, rawer and started to bleed. Was that pus? I kept being told the pain would pass. Meanwhile, I was steadily imbibing my fruit squash and felt as though my bladder would actually explode with how full I was. I timidly asked a few times why I felt so desperate to wee. I was told I had a catheter in, that it wasn't possible to wee normally at the moment. I texted my husband. FaceTimed him. Hours passed and while watching his newborn son fuss over the tiny phone screen, he noticed me wincing and asked what was going on. I explained that I felt like I was literally bursting with wee.

'Tell someone, Kim.'

I explained it wasn't that easy. I needed to turn and reach up for the CALL button each time and with my surgical wound, I was inflexible. When they did come, they just told me I was fine. I sighed and tried one more time. The nurse huffed, not acknowledging me, but reset the CALL button to stop the shrill ring. She looked down at me.

'I feel like I'm going to wee myself,' I confessed with a blush.

Sighing, she rounded the bed to look under the sheet for where my catheter bag was hanging.

'That's not possible, you have a cathet— oh.'

I whipped my head in her direction. She looked slightly sheepish and explained she'd get someone to remove the catheter so I could use the toilet. It turned out my bag hadn't been changed and there was nowhere for any more of my squash to go! I'm not a doctor or nurse and have no medical training, but didn't that mean the only way was up? As in, it was starting to go back up inside of me?

More public humiliation as the catheter was removed; they had to deflate the tiny balloon inside me that was anchoring the tube and pull it out. After this, I checked my son, who was unceremoniously wheeled back in and underwhelmingly reunited with me. I asked someone to keep an eye on him and readied myself for one of the greatest challenges of my life. No, not keeping the ever-unravelling fabric of my mind together. Not 'pushing past' the agonising first stages of breastfeeding, not walking unsteadily with stitches holding several layers of me closed. Not even the pain and discomfort of almost being able to feel my womb trying to shrink back down to size. No, it was time for the First Poo.

The end product would need to be examined by a nurse. So not only was I terrified that my internal organs would fall out along with it but *it* would have to be carefully retrieved for scrutiny.

Phase One, The Descent: I collected the disposable cardboard bed pan and headed into the toilet. I felt as weak as a kitten: pale, depleted and unsteady on my feet. I glanced at the toilet. My latest adversary. How was I going to do this? With no basic control over my abdominal muscles that usually helped me sit and stand with ease, how would I even lower myself to perch on the damn thing? I placed the paper commode on the floor. Now I needed to focus on the problem in front of me. I slowly turned and started to reverse, gathering up my nightie and lowering myself down. Usual rules don't apply during battle, so I put my hands directly on the toilet seat rim and took as much weight in my shaky arms as I possibly could. I almost fell the rest of the way, landing with a wince but at least I was back on terra firma. Sort of.

Phase Two, The Retrieval: Shit! Rookie error, I thought, as I realised my mistake. I'd left the bedpan on the floor. The hospital toilet was a little higher off the ground than normal, to aid patients with decreased mobility, I'd guess, so now I had to bend over the famously neat five-inch wound just below my pelvis that I was meant to be so enamoured with and fawn over its bikini-compatibility. That was fuck-all comfort right now. It was excruciating. My brow was sweaty and there was a slight tremor in my body. I felt like I was defusing a bomb rather than scooping down to pick up a paper bowl to shit in. My fingertips grazed it. Nearly there. One finger became two and as I dragged it towards me, I felt elated that I could finally grasp it with some purchase and slowly begin my ascent. Although now I was one hand short if I stumbled. I made it back up to sitting, dumping the receptacle in my lap to catch my breath before moving on to a dumping of another kind. I took a few steadying breaths. Shifting my weight onto one bum cheek, I tried to manoeuvre the bowl beneath me, between my legs, hovering above the water at the bottom of the stained bowl. I was ready.

Phase Three, The Push: The final push. When you normally go for a poo, you sit down, your brain tells your butt you're ready (again, I'm not medically trained), you engage a few muscles and gently push the parcel out. Wipe, flush and job's a good 'un. Now, I had to actively engage those muscles that felt so battered and bruised I could hardly keep from gasping. Even with a slight push, it felt as though my stitches would come undone, and my insides would fall out of my arse. I was terrified. This must be what death is like. No one can do it for you. No one can feel your fear. They're not on this one-way journey with you. My mind went to the first moon landing. While everyone was gushing over Armstrong and Aldrin, no one spared a thought for Michael Collins back in the lunar module. He later earned the moniker 'the loneliest man in the universe'. Buzz and Neil had each other for their moonwalk. Every other human being in existence was safely back on Planet Earth some 240,000 miles away. But he was on his tod, holding down the fort. That's how I felt now. The Loneliest Poo-er in the Universe.

There was some movement, shit – here it came, literally! I braced myself, precariously holding the rough cardboard container in place with an unnatural twist to my body. I just needed to get the head out, that was the tough bit, then the rest would follow. Like childbirth. Except I hadn't done that bit. I thought I'd got away with it, but the universe seemed to be having the last laugh. I imagined birthing a giant brown turd, having it swaddled in a John Lewis blanket and holding it lovingly to my bosom for those posed Instagram candids.

It was coming, it was coming! Then ... The Eagle Had Landed.

I think I caught it; I didn't hear the tell-tale splash, at any rate. I weaved my arm out from under me and there she was. Huh, there was some pee floating in there too. Was that okay? Could they run their highly technical lab tests without that contaminating the evidence? Having learned my lesson, I placed the bowl up on the cistern, did an absolutely shoddy at best job of wiping and steadily pushed to my feet. Giant nappy back in place, because *of course* there was a nappy involved, and pulled my pink, checkered nightshirt back into place. Like a lady. Keeping a side eye on The Poo, I washed up and then tentatively headed to the door with this precious, hard-won quarry in my quivering hands. I was exhausted.

I opened the door, looking for the nurse who should have

been waiting for me. The doorway was empty. Um, what should I do? I poked my head out into the corridor and saw she had wandered over to the main desk to chat with her colleagues. Fair enough, seeing as I had probably been in there for an hour. I gave a meek 'excuse me?', which shockingly she didn't hear, and decided there was nothing for it as I started heading towards her with a less than steely conviction. Don't mind me! I'm just a totally normal woman carrying her poo around in public, but if I could pass this test, then I could go home and back to my normal life. I'd feel lighter (literally), I'd feel like a mother, I'd feel . . . anything but this thick, cloying mass of darkness that was descending. Thankfully, she spotted me and met me halfway. I blushed and handed it to her. She looked down for possibly one-tenth of a millisecond, brought her face back to me and said, 'Great.' She shot past me, went back into the toilet I'd just vacated and, seconds later, I heard the flush. She hadn't? Had she? She can't have? I thought she was going to 'bag it' *CSI*-style and it would be rushed to the lab for a multitude of highly scientific, totally unfathomable tests. But it appeared my Herculean effort had meant nothing. They'd just wanted to see *if* I could shit by myself, not discover the meaning of life. She reappeared.

'Right, let's get you back to bed!'

★

We'd been in hospital for three days now, and something was possessing me. Infecting me. I kept FaceTiming my husband so he could see us. He said it was weird at home all by himself. It was weird in hospital, too. I'd also spent the last three days and nights quietly sobbing to myself. I was overwhelmed, exhausted and something felt very wrong. When asked 'how are you this morning?', I would automatically respond, 'OK, thanks, how are you?' That would earn me a tick in the box for Mother's Mental Well-Being in my trusty maternity file, a file that would soon be 'misplaced' during my hospital stay, meaning I couldn't have pain relief.

Suffice to say, at this point I was not okay. I felt like I was floating in a void, unable to fully grasp anything tangible, but at the same time hypervigilant. Every noise, every movement spooked me. The sounds of my baby's cry ran through my body with a shiver. The cot next to the bed was higher than said bed, so reaching over to pick him up was agonising and lying him back down without waking him near impossible. I went through my backpack. A Kindle? Who the fuck did I think I was kidding? That I'd give birth to a baby and then indulge in a little recreational reading? This wasn't a spa break.

The three other women in the ward came and went, faces changing as they were discharged and allowed their freedom. Owing to yet more Covid rules, we were restricted to our ward, and I had to knock on the door even to be allowed out to pee, as buzzers were hard to reach with abdominal wounds, or were sometimes ignored. I couldn't go outside for fresh air because, ironically, that was just for smokers. The walls were closing in on me. The temperature must have been a steady thirty degrees because I had a permanent film of sweat covering my skin. I felt clammy and dirty. It reminded me of the time I was in Guadeloupe to film *Death in Paradise* a few years before. I remember having a shower in my hotel room, stepping onto the bathmat, drying myself with a towel and in under a minute I was soaked with sweat again. The humidity was unreal, and we had continuity problems because of it. My hair would get bigger and bigger throughout a scene. But I wasn't in the Caribbean now. I was in a run-down, horribly clinical ward in a hospital in the middle of a housing estate in Merthyr.

I'd had my baby and while I was inundated with wonderful and well-intentioned messages, I felt the lowest I'd ever felt. Each text was a tiny dagger to my already hurting heart. I hated this. Did that make me a bad mum? I stared at my son's face for hours at a time, trying to feel the connection I was sure *must* be there. I took cute pictures and had a rolling WhatsApp conversation with my husband, who was stuck at home alone, unable to visit now the baby was on the ward with me. He made me laugh even through tears. He told me it was all going to be okay. He kept calling me Kimbo, which is how I knew I must be a mess.

★

Time meant nothing in there. The days and nights blended into a scheduled blob and revolved around doctors' rounds and nurses' observations. There was an almost laughable set-up where I and the baby needed to have our observations taken every four hours, but instead of coinciding them, we were split into a sleep-deprived, staggered routine. Mine were done at 8pm, 12am and 4am, and the baby's at 10pm, 2am and 6am, which meant that between feeding, burping, changing, settling him and both of us falling back to sleep, the curtain was ripped open approximately ninety minutes later. It felt like a cruel game, or a psychiatric test I wasn't confident I was passing.

There was nothing to do but wait. I didn't want to put my headphones in to watch something on my iPad because what if the baby needed me and I couldn't hear him? I didn't want to be like the bellend across the way from me who just watched Instagram reels on full volume or the girl next to me who, bizarrely, just stayed on FaceTime with her boyfriend twenty-four hours a day, even while she slept. You could hear him pottering about or playing Fortnite while she snored.

So, we waited.

And we waited.

Every time we got nearer to a discharge decision, a rash would be spotted, or a temperature would spike, or we had to wait for the next visit from the doctor, which if it didn't happen before a certain time meant an automatic rollover to the next day. I couldn't spend another night in this place. Until, finally, I was free. It felt like being emancipated from some subterranean cult. I was a mole-person being released back into the wild. I blinked at the pinkish-orange autumnal sunset, breathed in the slightly chilled, yet first real fresh air in days, and saw my husband walking towards me from the car park. It felt like not only had the season changed since I entered this building but the whole world, too.

4

The Fourth Trimester

(Or Death Becomes Her)

There is this theory called the Fourth Trimester. It's the first three months after birth and should be treated as a sacred and healing time, allowing your mind, body and soul to catch up with this monumental shift in your life. Yeah, I hadn't heard much about it either. Turns out it's REALLY fucking important. I blame rom-coms. Well, specifically the rom-com sequel because we all know the first movie ends with the wedding, leaving them to live happily ever after. Except, they miss out the bit where you have a huge comedown after spending a year planning, stressing, deciding and gearing up to the climax of your love story and then it's over and it's just, what? A normal Monday now? Not to mention having to become some sort of bureaucratic genius to change your last name on every document. About halfway through you morph into an anti-patriarchal feminist zealot when altering your surname just becomes too much of a ball ache.

The sequel is always 'having the baby' – the goofy romantic fun of making the baby (but without the IVF shag schedules), then the ever-growing bump with the decorating-of-the-nursery montage shoehorned in. The lovers playfully flick paint at each other. The woman is almost certainly in designer dungarees. Pro tip: you won't go inside that nursery for the next six months – other than to dump piles of clean clothes or in a frantic midnight scramble for a spare nappy. So, don't stress about it. Again, after the comedic climax of racing to the hospital and the female protagonist swearing her head off until a baby wails, the new mother (see: fully made-up Hollywood actress) has a soft sheen of sweat on her dainty brow as she's handed her newborn and is all smiles as she falls instantly in love. Then it's all dressing in white and lattes in the park with her mum friends while she 'enjoys' this new chapter.

For the next few months, there was no dressing in white without it immediately being doused in bodily fluids. Vaginal gunk, blood, milk, sick, shit, piss – it was a full medieval smorgasbord. I started to live with a cloth permanently draped on my shoulder. Admittedly, I gave birth in a pandemic (not recommended), so meeting for a coffee with mates involved either a measuring tape or a fine.

The day after we arrived home, Wales was plunged into what the Senedd (Welsh parliament) called a 'firebreak' in order to differentiate itself from Westminster (the British government), which was labelling it a 'circuit breaker'. Somewhere at the back of my mind, I mused that they sounded like the shit Gerard Butler films you find late at night on Amazon Prime. What it essentially meant was that the country was in quarantine and, as new parents, with an already shaky start, we could receive no visitors or benefit from any family help. The day after this, the clocks went back for Daylight Saving, so maybe it wasn't all in my head that I was plummeting into both a darkness and an isolation, the likes of which I'd never known. Were we all in this together? Judging by the later discovered Partygate, apparently not. First Minister of Wales, Mark Drakeford, would later tell a Covid inquiry that the local lockdowns of autumn 2020 were 'a failed experiment'. One where new mothers and their babies were the powerless guinea pigs. Glad we could be of service.

★

The truth was, I was finding this whole motherhood thing far tougher and more disturbing than I could ever have imagined. I wasn't taking to it like a duck to water, like everyone told me I would. I'd been a really hands-on aunty to my nephews and nieces, and had always thought it would be just a hop, skip and a jump to being a mum. Only now there was no reprieve, no respite – the buck stopped firmly with me. My decisions kept my baby happy and healthy and if I made the smallest mistake – not using the right blanket, not giving him enough milk – he could die and it would be all my fault. I could imagine it now: my husband would try to stand by me but the media attention would be too great. The court case too brutal. The strain on our marriage, no matter how much he loved me, couldn't survive me killing his son. No matter how unintentional.

I second- and third-guessed every micro-decision all day long. Could I go to the toilet for two minutes if he was safe in his Moses basket? What if something happened and he got trapped under a muslin and suffocated, or our dog suddenly attacked him and I didn't get there in time? No, it was best to take him with me. But then, are you allowed to pee in front of a minor? What are the rules on that? Is it okay if it's *your* kid? I would turn him away from me, so he couldn't see, not allowing the reality that not only was I his mother but his eyesight hadn't even fully formed yet. I couldn't even turn my back on him in bed while he was peacefully sleeping in his cot to my right, even though I'd been in the same uncomfortable position for hours. Did turning away from him mean I didn't love him? I couldn't be sure, so I wouldn't move a muscle, lying there quiet, still and in pain, but too scared to close my eyes. Then finally he would stir for a feed or a change, and another chance to sleep was gone.

I was tearful and in a lot of pain during those first days and weeks, and I could not stop thinking about terrible, terrible things – the worst things I could imagine happening to him or going wrong. Where was this all coming from? I couldn't shake it off, even though I physically tried to do just that: literally shaking my head to rid myself of these abhorrent thoughts and images. I was like a walking etch-a-sketch.

I didn't trust anything around me. My own senses were no longer reliable. I'd read some pseudo-anthropological meme on the internet that suggested the reason why babies usually looked like the father when their born was simply so that 'in the wild', they world recognise something of their gene pool in the offspring and stay. Most babies I knew always started out looking like the dad – it always seemed unfair after the woman had just done all the hard work. But my baby didn't look like my husband. He looked just like me. Or male members of my family and it threw me. What if he wasn't my husband's baby? Oh my god! What would I do?

This is ludicrous for two very salient reasons 1) we had done IVF and 2) my husband was the only man I had ever slept with, so unless there was a mix up in the lab, there was no rational thinking behind me confessing to my husband that *maybe* I'd cheated without remembering and we should do a paternity test for the bargain price of £99. I framed it as though it was a win-win. I knew he would love him either way but we'd have concrete proof of his biological link to this tiny baby or the fertility clinic would owe us a lot of money! He looked at me like I was insane. Guess I was. But it was a tangible example of how I couldn't stop trying to solve problems that didn't exist and profoundly distressing myself in the process. Nothing I did felt good enough, even though I was trying my absolute best. It got so bad that I considered signing over parental rights to my husband – you know, if it was his baby after all. It would be for the best. I shouldn't be allowed to make decisions; I wasn't in my right mind. I just couldn't move away from the idea that I was a bad person somehow and I was being punished for it. This mind of mine, constantly looking for irrefutable evidence of my innate badness, never seemed to take any of the victories into account. My son was growing and flourishing. His development was more or less on track and he was happy. He was loved and protected, even if I mistakenly thought I was keeping him protected from me. My heart would swell with every new facial expression, every newly perfected fine motor skill, every bubbly laugh and eventually every stumbled step and precious new word. But with the swells came the darkness, where my spirit felt as if it were being swamped by a thick black tar of self-disdain.

It wasn't like I'd never failed before, but if I failed at this, the consequences were dire. I could kill my baby. Everything made me feel like I was flunking motherhood. If someone saw him in stained baby clothes, they could speculate I wasn't coping. If someone smelt he'd done a poo before I did, they'd deliberate that I wasn't paying close enough attention. If he cried in my arms and someone swooped in to take him from me and he immediately stopped, it could only be because he sensed my evil. It was exhausting. I wasn't 'loving every minute' like I was supposed to. I wasn't even enjoying the nice bits. All my life I had tried to mitigate failure; why did I have to finally fall short now and at this?

Our time in the hospital had me convinced my baby would be taken from me. The sword of Damocles hung over us, and the anticipation was slowly killing me. I'd heard of the so-called baby blues and hoped that was all this was. Give it another week or so, I thought, and I'll be over the hump and can slide into that blissful baby bubble everyone told me so much about.

★

Here's where I should probably come clean and tell you that this wasn't the first time my brain had acted like it was in some sort of fucked-up alternate reality.

Yes, I'd struggled with anxiety and self-doubt as a teenager and often felt like my brain didn't work in the same way as everyone else's, but in the summer before my third and final year at drama school, something happened that felt a bit more worrying.

I was in an RSC sponsored production of *The Comedy of Errors*. I remember I was the Courtesan and wore a skirt made of blue hula hoops. All very post-modern. We were performing in Stratford-upon-Avon, the birthplace of Shakespeare and the home of the Royal Shakespeare Company. As part of the festival we were involved with, our company got to see lots of other plays that were on. One humid afternoon, during One of the Kings: Part Seventy-Five, we were into the third hour and my mind, understandably, started to wander. A thought popped into my head. An off-colour, unwanted sexual image that disturbed me and for some reason, I couldn't let go of. A nonsense train of thought had led me to this image and now I was stuck with it, replaying it over and over.

I couldn't shake the fact that I'd had this thought in the first place. It was a fleeting, nano-second image of a family member doing something gross and it repeated on a loop in my mind as I tried to stop it, or change it, or gauge what reaction I was having to it. I left that theatre shaken. Inconsolable, I rang my husband (who at that point was still my boyfriend) and tried to explain what had just happened. It's like I was fine one moment and broken the next. It felt that binary. For the rest of the week, I hardly ate or slept. I took myself away from the group when I felt I couldn't hold it together and faked it through smiles when I couldn't escape company.

Then I remembered that I had run two contraceptive pill packets together, as my costume was quite revealing and I didn't want to be on my period when performing at the Globe (see earlier re tampons). Perhaps it was something to do with that. I called my GP surgery back home and pleaded with the receptionist to let me talk to the doctor. When she informed me there was no one available, I asked her if she knew if the pill could have adverse effects. I'd been on it for a couple of years, so it would be unusual for something to happen at this point. She bumbled through an 'I'm not sure, love, sorry' before I was left holding my old brick of a mobile phone and feeling so lost, and scared that I was some kind of monster, even though I didn't want to be.

Was I a sexual deviant? I didn't think so; I loved my boyfriend and was hugely attracted to him, but why would an errant thought of that nature explode into my consciousness if it didn't mean anything? Was I into incest? Children? Animals? Inanimate objects? I didn't like the thought; even now my face grimaces. But what could it mean? What if it was a memory I had suppressed? What if it was a fantasy? I hated it – but did I? I just wanted it to STOP.

My dad attended our final performance. I'd had to find some forgotten corner of this famous theatre and attempt to get my breathing under control. Instead of marvelling that I was treading these hallowed boards, I had tunnel vision. At one point during the play, I would need to recite my monologue, and I knew if I stumbled over even one word it would be the final straw and, in front of hundreds of people and peers, I would fall apart. I delivered the monologue as directed. Nobody noticed a thing. Inside, I was shattering.

On the car journey home, I was so scared and ashamed to explain what had started all this, I just vaguely muttered something about feeling low and thinking bad thoughts. Dad drove me home to Wales where I just wanted to forget this had ever happened. I think he sensed not to push too far with his questions as I was so visibly upset. Once I'd reassured him that nothing had happened to me – I can only imagine what must run through a father's mind when his daughter departs for a trip full of excitement and comes back a shell of her former self – the rest of the drive was conducted in silence. Not like us at all. We're chatterers when we're together. We gossip and joke and generally talk about everything and nothing. But I couldn't. I felt disgusting and contaminated with 'bad thoughts' and wanted the car seat beneath me to swallow me whole.

I told my boyfriend everything. I confessed to every 'bad

thought' I'd EVER had. Compulsively. I was viewing the world differently, checking my responses to the people around me. Trying to assure myself I hadn't done anything inappropriate. What would happen if anyone found out? What would happen to me when my true nature was revealed? I wanted to be a good person. I had always tried my best to be a good person. Had it all been a lie? My boyfriend assured me it was just a weird blip, an errant thought, everyone had them, he had them all the time. But why was it affecting me so profoundly, yet he could shrug it off? He brushed it off with an 'everyone has accidentally thought of their nan during a wank' placation. I'm paraphrasing.

When I came to think of it, however, I did have weird impulses sometimes. Every time I travelled to London and stood waiting for the tube at Victoria Station, for example, I'd always had this urge to duck my head out as the train roared past. What would that be like? Would I feel anything? Or would it be over in an instant? The poor driver though. Who cleans the windscreen? I didn't want to actually do it, of course, so I could easily shrug it off. Ah ha! Yet more evidence that THIS alarming, unshakable thought must be more significant. 'You're overthinking it, Kim,' my boyfriend said, 'it doesn't mean anything.'

Maybe he was right, but for the next few months I was beside myself. He held me through inconsolable crying and chronic doubt as I tried to rehearse for my next role as Abigail in *The Crucible*. I quickly learnt how to channel all that emotion into something more useful performance-wise but that only gets you so far.

As a result of this 'episode', I went to the doctor. I was diagnosed with the joyfully vague title of generalised anxiety disorder

(GAD), which basically meant I was anxious but no one knew why. I remember my first foray into therapy – three sessions with a very nice lady who drew a cup on a piece of paper. Most people's cups were only a third full much of the time, she explained, so whenever the stress tap was inevitably turned on, they had room in their cup to deal with it. My cup was already full, so tap stress had nowhere to go. My cup did indeed runneth over, except that the 'cup' was my young mind and the 'tap' was stuck in the ON position, the overflow an unknowable quantity of ambiguous anxiety and general bad thinking. I felt like calling a plumber. All I could picture was Mario doing his little jump in the air while pixelated tears poured out the side of his face.

It was also why, during my pregnancy, I had self-referred to Perinatal Mental Health via my midwife. I'd felt great during this time; I'd come a long way since my early twenties and that previous episode in Stratford-upon-Avon at the Royal Shakespeare Theatre and knew much more about myself and how my brain worked, but it was a precautionary measure so that I could be monitored. It had seemed like the sensible thing to do.

And it was why now, as I turned to my husband, tears in freefall, holding our weeks-old baby, I could simply say 'it's happening again' and he instantly understood. It was fine, he said. We'd go to the doctor. It would all be fine. My GP and the practice nurse (an old friend of ours) knew my history, knew me and how pragmatic I was about my mental health and immediately understood the gravity of the situation. Quickly my antidepressants were upped and Perinatal Mental Health were looped in.

Baby blues conjure such a soft, Beatrix Potter-like idea of a woman so overwhelmed with happiness that the silly mare can't get a handle on herself. But there was nothing cosy or brimming with delight about what was unfurling in my eclipsing mind. I consoled myself that at least my body was healing rapidly and I was keeping relatively active. If I can't be of use mentally, I thought, then goddammit, I would be so physically capable they'd want to use me as a case study for speedy post-operative bounce back. I concentrated on keeping up with all feeds, changes and baby-related tasks. I had to do it all or I'd be failing. My hope was that in the comfort and familiarity of my own home, breastfeeding and other such literal teething troubles would be easier. Less pressurised without an audience.

*

We settled into a kind of hapless routine, on a four-hourly basis of feeds, changes, winding, repeat. But there was no reprieve in how on edge I was. Darting eyes, racing heart, pure liquid dread whenever I looked at the little bundle of responsibility, I was terrified would die on my watch. And there was no end in sight to the boundless back-rubbing trying to elicit that elusive burp. Or fart. Any expulsion of air from his tiny body would do, as it meant the shrill screams would stop and while my husband was also affected by the unrelenting squawks, he wasn't paralysed with fear over them. Me, it was like my body was almost trying to repel the sound. Each clawing wail seemed to alter me on a molecular level. This didn't bode well as I'd heard that babies cry. A lot. Still, we marvelled at our son's cherubic face, received warm wishes and gifts from friends and family and took copious amounts of pictures with him in cute, novelty outfits doing cute, involuntary movements we were adamant were intentional and pointed toward a genius beyond his age.

But something was just plain wrong.

My world was off its axis, and I just didn't know if this was normal or not. My house looked the same but felt off, crooked and unnerving. I looked at my son, at his cloudy grey-green eyes, so big and innocent, and I found myself rubbing my chest to relieve my hurting heart. I wasn't sure I could do this. As this ominous feeling continued to loom, outwardly I appeared to be nailing it. I put make-up on and got dressed every morning – even though we were essentially confined to four walls – because God forbid the health visitor should turn up and think I'm not coping. I ate but tasted nothing. I watched Netflix with unseeing eyes. I slept for short bursts but didn't really rest. I could always feel my husband side-eyeing me, watching closely, noticing that I was clearly not myself. Under his knowing scrutiny, I was unsuccessful at putting up a front. A 'fake it till you make it' mentality that wasn't quite coming up with the goods.

The scary, disgusting thoughts were coming thicker and faster, and I was losing the battle to prevent the deluge. They were also getting more violent and horribly sexual, and I could feel my mind's defences weakening. I didn't yet know that this had a name – Intrusive Thoughts – and I was unaware that 98 per cent of new parents report having them. I just knew that I was frantically treading water, gasping for air as I held my baby above the waves while trying to kick free of the strong grasp some dark entity had on my ankles. Pulling me down. Down, down. I embraced my baby tightly on our sofa and so wanted to enjoy this time. With love and fear in my eyes, I looked down at him and craved feeling that burst of overwhelming joy. I wanted to remember who I was 'before' but I couldn't quite reach it. I couldn't seem to tap into those memories, and it felt wrong somehow to try and create new ones under this veil.

The thoughts would start out reasonable enough. The fear largely centred around one, all-consuming question – was he safe? That would then terrifyingly morph into – is he safe from me? And what I couldn't get past was that I was having to ask this question in the first place. It must have meant something. It must. But what? When I was changing him, I'd worry that he could roll and fall onto the hard kitchen tile. Maybe I should put the changing mat on the floor and take gravity out of the equation? But what if the dog walked over him and scarred him for life with her claws? When I was breastfeeding him, I'd worry if he was getting enough. I couldn't tell; I didn't have transparent boobs. If I was bottle-feeding him, I'd worry if the milk was the right temperature. Did using this intermediary vessel to facilitate his feeding mean we wouldn't bond as well as if he was EBF (Exclusively Breast-Fed)? Possibly, according to some forums on Mumsnet. If I was bathing him, I'd wonder if the water was too hot or too deep. Why was he crying? Was the water hurting him? When he was in his pram, I'd worry if he was warm enough. These were perfectly legitimate concerns for a nervous new parent, of course, but they didn't end there. They kept extrapolating out, becoming wilder and even more nonsensical to others but wholly logical and valid to my ever-eddying mind. Worrying if his bath was the right depth or temperature quickly mutated into him drowning and me being too shocked to jump into action and stop it. Being warm enough in his pram on a winter's walk would mushroom out into him being smothered by blankets or dying of hypothermia because I got something wrong. Then I would have to push his cold, blue little body home and explain to my husband what I'd done.

My imagination knew no bounds. It was a murky and obscure

thought-soup of threat, peril and morbidity. Someone had ordered his kidnapping on the dark web, his milk powder was contaminated with anthrax, that little rash that had popped up was meningitis but was an as-yet-unknown strain that tricks you by disappearing under a glass rolled on the skin. What if a paedophile ring got their hands on him while we were out shopping or at the park? What would they do to him? I locked the doors, checked for secret cameras, kept monitoring his little body for signs of disease, tried some of his milk on the tip of my tongue like a medieval royal taster allowing any poison to kill me first. Was that a gurgle or was he gasping for breath? When I had put every safety barrier in place, the only unknown quantity was an exhausted, hormonal, different *me* who I didn't know and could no longer trust. Policing my mind and body for any hint of a red flag became my driving force and sole purpose in this new existence.

And I was entirely ashamed of myself for it.

Everything was corrupted. My thinking was skewed. I was living in the Upside Down from *Stranger Things*, a thick, black tar rolling over every aspect of my life, suffocating the life out of it. I took a posed, smiling selfie with my newborn son in my favourite, battered pink sweatshirt. Complete with artificial rosy cheeks and lips, I posted it to my private, friends and family only, Facebook – and burst into tears. With every new 'like', I cried harder. I hated this new reality and, with every moment I wished I could just go back, my heart sank at the notion that would mean not having him here. What kind of a mother wishes for that? I must be a monster. I began to convince myself that this was simply the trade-off. Nothing in life truly comes for free. For him to be here – happy and healthy – just meant

I couldn't be. It was a cruel curse but one I was glad to bear as the lesser of two evils. Either I was miserable, or my baby would be. I believed this self-imposed rule so emphatically that it restored my conviction to carry on. He would thrive if I could just survive.

I stared at my naked body in the mirror. Huge brown nipples, so much larger than normal, almost like each tit was wearing a beanie. Trailing my gaze downwards, my comforting, firm bump was now a flaccid void. The C-section scar — the one I should marvel over — was sore yet protected with a white, self-adhesive bandage. My face was sunken and gaunt. My eyes, only one week previously bright chocolate orbs brimming with excitement, were now a dull, lifeless, shitty brown.

I tried so desperately to push past it. To be normal. We met with some family in Barry Sidings, a lovely countryside park with playground and café, formerly an old railway storage area and on the direct line from Pontypridd to Barry Docks for precious coal to be exported around the world. My gorgeous newborn, wrapped in layers of wool to ward off the biting, cold weather, was doted on by relatives getting to see him properly for the first time, albeit from a distance. I had a flat white in my hand, a cute bobble hat on my head, even some lipstick and I thought, am I doing it? Am I the Instagram mum of my stylish dreams pushing my buggy around and 'bouncing back'? To the casual observer, maybe. But inside, I was dimming by the minute. I felt suffocated and inexorably broken. I couldn't stop checking that his miniature face wasn't covered over by a blanket or that he hadn't frozen to death in the last few minutes. My shrewd sister-in-law noticed. She'd obviously been watching me for a while.

She sidled up to me with a sympathetic smile.

'You can't stop checking on him, can you?'

'No,' I admitted and tried to laugh it off as the stereotypical, frazzled new mum, but my body was fizzing with the need to peer into the pram one more time. To get another fix, another micro-dose of short-lived relief. She told me it was normal, which I'm sure it was, but the constant demand to physically check he was alive was raking over my skin like a horde of cockroaches. (Sidenote: I just looked this up as I enjoy collective nouns, and a group of cockroaches is actually called an intrusion. How apt.)

★

In amongst the mental torment was a flurry of corporeal excruciations. My boobs were throbbing and beyond sore. They became hot to the touch and even a cotton T-shirt brushing against them was too much. I started to get a fever and, after calling the GP surgery, thinking they'd brush me off, I was told to come straight in. I wasn't supposed to drive as I wasn't out of the C-section woods, but if my husband drove me then we'd have to wake the baby, who'd only just dropped off. My husband pleaded with me, but I told him I'd be there and back in no time, and it would be easier without lugging the baby and all necessary accoutrements out into the dark, blustery afternoon. 'And I could do with five minutes to myself.' He relented.

I didn't wear a seat belt.

Me, a stickler for the rules. A que-sera-sera sensation settled over me. I wasn't going to instigate a car crash but if I got into one, so what? I almost shrugged. Would that be such a bad thing? It was almost as if fate was in the empty passenger seat beside me, Thelma and Louise style.

An old schoolfriend was the doctor on-call – welcome to small town living. She was so happy to see me and asked about the baby. She'd attended my baby shower only a little while ago. It had been a beautiful, crisp September afternoon. My friends had thrown a surprise shower in the garden, as you could only meet outside. I'd been so delighted to see everyone; for some, the first time seeing me pregnant, and I'd just drunk it all in. The balloons, the sickly-sweet zero per cent Prosecco, the tiny crustless sandwiches and the absolute mountain of gifts. Gosh, our little boy was going to be surrounded by so much love, and I was glowing with affection for such good friends and the future to come. Now, topless in a blanched, fluorescent-lit doctor's surgery being told I have mastitis and needed antibiotics, I couldn't see that glow for dust.

It was the middle of the night, and I was topless, once again. My tits were hovering over a glass mixing bowl filled with steamy, boiling water and I was awkwardly dunking one in, desperate to alleviate the pressure of engorgement and blocked milk ducts. The baby started crying from our bedroom; my husband must have woken up as I heard 'Kim, can you do a bottle?' being stage-whispered down the stairs. I felt wrung-out. So tired, I wasn't even sleepy, just stupefied. And the guilt of not 'enjoying every minute' was eating away at me. An insidious woodworm. Shoulders slumped, I dried off my chest with a tea towel and made a bottle before trudging back upstairs. Back to it.

★

I ventured out to the supermarket. I'd always found supermarkets a sort of cathedral, the white noise of shoppers, announcements and trundling trolleys very calming. I liked to go by myself and slowly browse. I liked that no one bothered me. I could breathe there. So, I went solo to the supermarket with my weeks' old baby. I walked around in a delirious daze, meandering from fruit and veg to canned goods, not remotely remembering what we needed. I generally like to push the trolley down the central aisle, park it and run down each side aisle to grab what I need in the supermarket. I've always done this. I left the trolley and wandered away to grab some milk. I was just getting to the one I needed – four pints, green top – and then I remembered: there's a baby in my trolley. For about ten seconds I'd forgotten my son's entire existence. Never mind that this was my first post-birth supermarket trip, and I'd just acted out of habit. Never mind that the trolley was only twenty feet away from me the entire time. Never mind that he was fast asleep and didn't register my absence. I'd forgotten my son existed.

And then it all came crashing back in: the pain and fear of the past weeks, the birth, the hellish hospital stay and my total inability to land back into my own life now that I was a mother, all hit me like an articulated lorry. I dashed back to him. Checked he wasn't hurt or injured, that he wasn't in any distress. Did someone touch him while my back was turned? How could I forget him like that? What kind of a person, what kind of a mother, forgets that she has a baby with her? I remembered reading an article once about a woman in America who had accidentally left her baby inside a car for hours. She was sleep-deprived and forgot the baby was in the back seat asleep while she popped into work. The baby died from the heat. I knew we were headed into winter, but what if I did that and he froze to death all alone in the back of my car? This was yet more proof that I couldn't let my guard down for a millisecond. What if someone had just walked off with the trolley and he'd been raised by another family, leaving us to spend the rest of our lives searching for him? What if they'd hurt him, what if they'd wanted to do terrible things to my precious little boy? I grabbed him from the inbuilt baby seat in the trolley and rushed out of the shop.

When I got home, I confessed the terrible thing I'd done to my husband in floods of tears. He assured me that I was just tired, I was still in shock from the birth, it had only been a few seconds and I'd never gone shopping with my own baby before. It was just an oversight. Nothing had happened. I was a good person, and I needed to stop beating myself up. I heard none of it. And I'd forgotten to buy the milk.

★

Supermarkets were a running theme. I suppose, because of Covid, they were one of the few places people could socialise. Not long after this, I got back on the horse and ventured out to the shops again. I'd even made it as far as the check-out when an older lady drifted over and asked the standard 'how old?', not looking at me but down at my little bundle of joy. He was in the built-in baby trolley seat looking out at us, wide-eyed, and after I had answered however many weeks, she then, out of nowhere, remarked, 'It's terrible, isn't it, what some people do to them?'

It was like that famous zoom moment in *Jaws*. My world got bigger and smaller at the exact same time. It felt like I was the only person in the room while also feeling crowded and boxed in. What? Why would she say that? Is she bad? Does she think I'm bad? Is the world as dark and bad as my brain is insisting it could be? I had the world's quietest panic attack, nothing showing outwardly but I may as well have had a shot of cold, liquid, medical-grade anxiety jabbed into my spine. After packing and paying, I darted to the car once again. What the hell was going on?

★

Slowly, the worse I looked, the more serene I felt, as though paying a physical penance for such horrendous visions in my mind was balancing the cosmic books somehow. If I was rotten to the core on the inside, it was only right that it should be reflected on the outside. I began to eat crap as a punishment. The nourishing green, leafy vegetables and fresh fruits of my pregnancy were long forgotten when getting a takeaway during the pandemic had become the norm. It was perfectly understandable for new parents to indulge in the odd pizza or Chinese takeaway amongst all the upheaval. But eating that stuff was making me feel a tangible disgust that was easier to focus on than the grotesque, almost chemical, breakdown that was occurring within my sad, battered mind. Just Eat was doing great business from me. I felt like I should have a Breakdown Loyalty Card: buy four stodgy curries and the fifth one comes with free poppadoms and a box of Kleenex for your snot and self-loathing.

Everything haunted me. Waking in the night to tend to my baby, I was transported to a shadowy TV drama where I was the villain, hovering above the cot with evil intent. Each time, I hoped it would be different but the first thing I'd do when I woke up would be to see if *it* had gone – *it* being the bad thoughts, but thinking of *it* negated that hope and perpetuated the cycle.

You know that unearthly space between sleep and coming fully awake, where things have the potential to be a dream before your consciousness is flooded with the day ahead or memories of yesterday? That place, that plain was where my sense of hope went to die each morning. Slowly. Death by a thousand cuts. I was being tortured by what *could be* and not what was. When that's your reality, it's a drawn-out yet direct hit to your heart. Soon I was shrouded in the thoughts of a thousand different ways I could ruin the most precious thing in my life, so completely, so utterly, that the fabric of my being was irrevocably shattered. I would shake on hearing his mobile play lullabies, the innocent sound so sinister to my ears. 'Twinkle, Twinkle, Little Star' had become the leitmotif of my own personal horror film. I dreaded bath times. Nappy changes. Feeds. I started to wish upon a star that I would never wake up when I *was* finally able to fall asleep.

The worst thing was that I didn't understand what was happening to me. I'd been fine a few weeks ago. Now, I couldn't focus on anything but the intense worry that something bad would happen to him. Every little cough was a life-threatening choke. Every gurgle, a first sign of cystic fibrosis. If I saw red in his eyes in a photograph, that was an undiscovered brain tumour. Same if the dog came sniffing around him as I fed on the sofa. Couldn't some dogs smell cancer? I thought I'd read that in *Take A Break* or *Woman's Own*. I was so overloaded by the sounds of having a baby in the house, I wanted to scream. But I didn't. I was quiet. So quiet, it was unnerving.

Weeks transitioned into months and on Christmas Eve – my favourite day of the year – I sat in our old, sage-green armchair, the one we'd bought from a charity shop years before for our first-ever home. I cradled my baby and watched *The Snowman*. I was desperately trying to create core memories for him as well as myself. I felt nothing but a melancholy so deep, I was drowning in despondency. This was one of those Richard Curtis-esque, life-affirming moments when the dream of becoming a mother had felt like it was slipping away during those years of infertility. But another tear spilt over and gently landed on his pastel blue blanket (a cellular one, lots of holes, so he couldn't suffocate) and I couldn't quite believe this was my life. It was a daily waking nightmare, one in which I second-guessed every touch or look with my own baby. I quietly shook with dread in the low glow of twinkly lights and the angelic melodies of Aled Jones. Except it wasn't Aled Jones. That was just for the charts. The film's soundtrack was sung by St Paul's Cathedral choirboy, Peter Auty. I wondered if it bums him out every time the festive season rolls around that he didn't get the recognition he deserves. I guessed the royalties must have kept a turkey on the table – that would console him, I reasoned.

I heard my husband's footfall in the hallway and wiped away all evidence of any weeping, but I wasn't fooling anyone. With a strong but soothing hand on my shoulder, he asked if I was okay. Just hormones, I said. And beseeched any higher power that might exist to make this true. The only other explanation was eternal damnation, but my heart was too broken to face that prospect just yet. My husband suggested I shouldn't sit in near darkness watching what he called the most 'wistful film ever' and I informed him it was tradition, whether I felt like it or not.

Christmas came and went. We got that photo as a family of three around the Christmas tree like I'd dreamt of the previous year, but I felt nothing of what I expected. It was hard to enjoy cutesy elf onesies and Baby's First Christmas joy when all I could see were visions of death and abuse. Every moment of my day flickered alongside this horror slideshow. Like that bit in *A Clockwork Orange* where his eyes are held open by metal pincers, forcing him to see the unseeable. Until finally, one January day – with a sprinkle of a medication change acting as a catalyst – it all became frighteningly crystal clear. I knew how it could finally, finally stop.

I was on a Welsh mountain in a wintry forest, everything

calm, my dog, Bob, running wild and free, when my upward march was brought to an abrupt halt. The thought slotted in so cleanly, so obviously, that I laughed out loud that it had taken me so long to arrive at the solution. I couldn't live like this for much longer. My son was just over three months old and as well as *it* not lifting, it had been getting heavier and darker, and I was moving further away from my reality.

I couldn't stop thinking. That was just science. For as long as I had a working brain, it would think, and I couldn't think my way out of this. I'd spent 8,640,000 seconds proving that rule. And my word, had I felt every nanosecond of that. It wouldn't stop when I slept because I either didn't sleep or had night terrors. It didn't cease even when I was sedated under strong medication. Then it just became a surreal montage of revolting mirages. There was only one way to make my brain stop. It was *so* elementary. If my body wasn't alive then my brain would die. My mind couldn't torture me, and I could be the most certain of all that I wouldn't be a danger or a burden to anyone I loved. A parasite can't survive on a dead host. As a lifelong deliberator, this was the easiest decision of my entire life. I would cease to exist, this would end, and my baby would be truly, one hundred per cent, beyond a shadow of a doubt, safe from me.

Okay, now we were cooking.

I felt lighter than I had in months. What was today? The 27th of January; the first of February would fall on a Monday. Perfect. I would do it this Sunday. End of the month, so my husband and son could start the week and the month afresh, rid of any encumbrance I'd been imposing on them. That gave me four days to get everything in order. I took my phone out and a selfie captured the moment. In time, my husband would find this image and understand it better than any explanation I could give. My pale, drawn, devastated face would say it all.

I felt renewed with a sense of purpose. So many plans to make and so little time. The where, the how, the what-after. I thought it through carefully and realised I could never allow my husband to find me. That would be too cruel. He didn't have the near-eidetic memory I did, but even he wouldn't be able to shake that tableau. Okay, how to make this as easy on everyone as possible? It wasn't the melodramatic, climactic thought process films and television would have you believe – there was a quiet, steely determination. It was almost clinical and such a relief after the torment of the past months. I had so much to get ready. This was my time to shine. Financially, emotionally, logistically, I wanted to make this as straightforward and as easy on everyone as possible.

I googled methods of suicide. In some other incarnation of myself, I thought how ludicrously far I had strayed from where all this had begun. Us, in love, just wanting to have a family. But that wasn't for now. Stupid Google didn't even show you means of self-annihilation, just The Samaritans' helpline number. Couldn't they see I was on a schedule? I checked the weather app on my phone. Snow was forecast on Sunday, D-Day. That was nice, I love snow. I was standing in a hillside copse and saw a sturdy tree with a good, thick branch extending out horizontally. Perfect. I knew we had rope in the garage. My father-in-law is a climber, and I was pretty sure he'd lent my husband ropes for transporting our Christmas tree on the roof of the car last month.

A plan was forming; it was neat, it was effective, and it was minimally impactive. If I hanged myself from this tree on a path through the mountainside that hardly anyone used and I called the emergency services just as I was going through with it, they'd send out seasoned professionals to find me. The fire or ambulance service people would have seen a dead body before, so I wouldn't be traumatising them. The chances of being happened upon by a passerby were minimal. I would have ID in my pocket, so my husband wouldn't have to identify me and this way, it'd be as efficient and pain-free as I could possibly make it. I'd have letters ready to explain to my husband and my dad, and one for my son when he was older.

I got home from that walk and my husband's Spidey senses were immediately heightened. I was calmer and happier than I'd been since before the birth. He was confused, I could see it. I told him the medication must be working. Little did I know it was doing the complete opposite – I was the walking, talking epitome of their small-print T&Cs. Antidepressants can cause a rapid, initial shift in serotonin levels and could disrupt other neurotransmitter systems or receptor subtypes, leading to paradoxical effects –like making you a hell of a lot worse before it starts to make you better.

I tried to arrange an online will and life insurance, but it turned out you can't collect on the insurance if the suicide is committed within the first twelve months after the policy is taken out. Clever bastards. Shit, no payday there then for my kith and kin. That was okay – I had savings, for self-employed tax purposes, but did dead people pay tax? Hmm, not sure. Add it to the list. They could sell the house – it would be theirs to do with as they wished. I thought of writing a letter for every birthday for my son's next eighteen birthdays but quickly concluded, what would I say past letter number ten? How do you guide a teenage boy from beyond the grave? Wear deodorant, use a condom, don't say 'I love you' unless you really mean it, watch *The Princess Bride* because it's brilliant and know, as the moon causes the tides, that I loved you so profoundly I would rather not be here than see a single hair on your head hurt.

It was that simple for me. They were mutually exclusive. It was me or him, and I chose him in every scenario.

I worked away in the background, making sure the council tax, energy provider and banking paperwork were at hand for afterwards. I wrote three letters. One for my husband, one for my father and finally one for my little boy. I knew that my son might be angry with me when he was older, thinking I'd left him behind, but if he could just see *why* I was doing this, that really, I was helping and that this was for the best.

I went for a bracing walk with my husband, the baby bundled up in the pram and we strolled amongst the bare trees, along a tarmacked path. I peeked at my husband as he chatted to me, taking him in, enjoying this last bit of time together. I smiled to myself that he didn't realise in just a few short days, things would be *so* much better. Just you wait and see.

Second spoiler: I didn't kill myself. My new medication evened out and I began to claw back to an even keel. The haze cleared and I came clean to my husband about a week later when realising how scarily close I'd come to something so definitive and so far away from who I really was. But I still spent every night lying between my husband on one side and my baby in the next-to-me crib on the other, petrified with fear and an anxiety so deeply ingrained that if I didn't keep an eye on myself every second of every day, the unthinkable could happen. It was then we realised this wasn't going anywhere. I needed more help.

5

Intrusive Thoughts

(Or Where Did You Go To, My Lovely?)

My grandmother would reportedly say, 'evil thinkers, evil doers'. I didn't know her very well, only meeting her briefly when I was seventeen, just before she passed away. She sounded like the loveliest, most kind-hearted lady, and I know my dad thought the world of her. This family idiom was often used in a consolatory capacity. That nasty person only accused you of that nasty thing because it's something their nasty minds would conjure up. It was meant to soothe you. But I would play that phrase over and over again, like a distant record player in the back of my mind, and truly wonder, 'Were evil thinkers, evil doers?' God, I hope not. But hoping isn't sure. Sure is sure. Better check myself again. Just to be sure.

At this point, I didn't know this vicious circle or pathological need for reassurance had a name. In fact, it would take months to find the end of this tangled ball of thought-string. Some brave, anonymous soul posted an account of their scary intrusive thoughts about their baby and feeling like they were living in a constant state of terror. It was the first description that resonated with me. I didn't know that those intrusions, which had been popping into my mind's eye since childhood, making me feel crazy, had an actual name. But while there was a groundswell of relief at recognising my symptoms, part of me was too scared to click on the link for more information. And that, my friend, is the evil genius of obsessive compulsive disorder, which after four months of hell, was what the internet was telling me I had. It makes you believe that asking for help, being honest and trying to learn more about the disorder, rather than your particular obsession within it, will be your downfall.

I told my GP that I didn't feel I was ticking the postnatal depression boxes, but this? This article was like someone had hijacked the livestream of my brain. She agreed that my symptoms fitted an OCD diagnosis, so we looped in Perinatal Mental Health.

As you'll have gathered, the biggest problem I was having was with intrusive thoughts, rumination and internal echolalia (the silent and involuntary repetition of words, sounds or phrases – a term I wouldn't learn for another four years, until my autism diagnosis). Although I'd struggled with this for much of my life – most dramatically in that theatre run in Stratford – I now knew what it was called. So much of my childhood slid into place like that last jigsaw piece. Why, for example, when I watched an episode of Poirot when I was eight years old, I couldn't stop thinking about it, or twisting it about in my mind 24/7 for a couple of months afterwards. I could see and hear it so clearly. Over and over. No room for anything else. The only way I could sleep was to listen to a mixed cassette of different Christmas songs and feel some short relief in the familiarity of George Michael's 'Last Christmas'. When you're eight, you think it's magical or maybe a Roald Dahl Matilda mind trick thing?

INTRUSIVE THOUGHTS

Though now, I knew it wasn't harmless. It was fucking destructive. It would take an age, hard work and endless stumbles for me to realise that it didn't have to be.

One time, my husband had gone to work – his light beginning to dim under this intense pressure too - and I hadn't slept *again*. I was in old and dirty pyjamas that I think used to be white but were now a kind of comforting greige. I decided to have a shower. Monumental stuff! I could freshen up and wash away this all-consuming anxiety and depression and I would feel better. Then I could be a normal mum and go to the park with him or something. He would be okay in his baby bouncer on the floor just outside the shower cubicle, wouldn't he?

Suddenly, under the hot spray, my heart rate spiked, and I got that clawing feeling along my skin again. Was this okay? Were you allowed to be naked in front of a baby? Why was I making him watch? I thought I'd turned him to face me so I could keep an eye on him, but what if something more sinister was going on? What if this was sexually inappropriate? My skin was heating up and I didn't know where to look. I wanted to crawl out of my own skin to make this feeling stop. I cut the shower off, not even having finished rinsing out the shampoo, and raced to get dressed. Still wet from the shower, suds still in my knotted hair.

Another time, I was looking down at my little guy wearing a cowboy onesie, something I had been so excited to buy when I was pregnant, envisioning my future baby in it. And here he was, perfect and healthy and *here*. The five-year heartache of every period signalling I wasn't pregnant had melted away because I finally had everything I'd ever wanted.

I was staring down at him and taking pictures. Partly because

I wanted to – *but why, Kimberley?* my brain asked. *Why do you want to take photographs of your baby? What are you going to do with them?* – and partly because I didn't feel present, and I genuinely wanted something by which to remember these moments I knew were passing me by. I was gazing, I was looking, I was checking how my body was reacting, I was looking at my hands to make sure they weren't doing anything inappropriate – and then he started to get grizzly. He needed feeding. I hated this bit. A few months in and breastfeeding was still beyond painful.

I scooped him up and sat on his bedroom floor facing the mirrored wardrobe, glancing around this nursery we had so excitedly painted and decorated with a woodland theme. No one said we were original, but I loved the forest near our home and spent a lot of time there walking Bobbie in between fertility tests and treatments, and being let out for our one hour of exercise a day during Covid restrictions, so it felt apt. Now, it all seemed sad and wistful and ruined. I wasn't doing this right. I wasn't getting any of it right. He was whining in my arms; I sighed and lifted up my top to breastfeed him. He struggled against me, he didn't want it, he was probably too used to the bottles of my expressed milk. I kept failing him. I just wanted to get this right.

I tried again, nipple-to-nose, and pushed it into his little suckling mouth but it hurt so much, and he began to really cry. I was essentially shoving my tit into some baby's mouth and I started to shake. I looked up and caught a glimpse of my reflection. The heating was on; I was wearing a blue woolly roll-neck jumper that was now unbearably hot. My body was so tense you could have snapped it like a breadstick. I was ready to explode and I realised that maybe this was what abuse looked

INTRUSIVE THOUGHTS

like. Was I making him do something inappropriate? Was I abusing my baby? Why was he crying? Why was *I* crying?

I pulled back aghast, my areola raw and agonisingly tender. I stood and placed the baby back in the cot. What had I done? What had I *just* done? Was this it? The irrevocable bad 'thing' that I couldn't take back? I stared down at him, appalled at myself. What should I do? I was sobbing uncontrollably. I raced downstairs with the idea of getting him a bottle but sank to the kitchen floor propped up against the cupboard door – like some shitty, badly acted Sunday evening TV drama. I wheezed through what was undoubtedly a panic attack as my mind fully and almost completely collapsed in on itself. I was an abuser, a child abuser. I didn't want to be a child abuser! Or was that just a lie I told myself to feel better? Had I been like this all along and giving birth had awoken the Kraken?

I wouldn't eat or interact. My husband called the emergency health visitor, and she came around – a nice lady I'd never laid eyes on before – and I didn't move the whole time she was there. I answered her questions robotically and later found out that when my husband showed her to the door, she told him, 'She's very unwell.' She told him I desperately needed to be sedated – I was dangerously sleep-deprived – I had barely slept for ten days straight – and was given an emergency prescription, which was hard to come by normally, but during Covid? Unheard of. He came back into the living room where I was so spaced out with exhaustion and lost to unrelenting, repulsive images that when he asked if he should ask his mam to pop round while he ran to the pharmacy, I just nodded. I'd been trying to hide it from our families for months, so this was a worrying sign for him that I'd truly given up.

My mother-in-law seemed to walk into the room only seconds later, but I know that can't be true. She hugged me and I cried. I said I was so sorry. Time lost all meaning. Again, it only seemed like moments later that my husband was handing me two pills and a glass of water. I didn't even ask, I just took them and swallowed. My mother-in-law stood up so they could chat about what to do next and within half a sentence when they turned back to ask me a question, I had keeled over on the couch. I went on to sleep in that exact spot for the next sixteen hours inside a hellish fever dream. But at least I was asleep.

★

Think of the most disturbing scene from a film that you can recall. One that doesn't quite leave your psyche even days later, one that made your skin crawl. Maybe you watched it at the IMAX, with Dolby Surround Sound and one of those old scratch 'n' sniff cards. On repeat. Then make the focus of that unstoppable tirade of disgusting images your tiny newborn baby. Now imagine being locked in a dark room where that scene plays on loop for minutes, hours, weeks, or in my case months, and eventually years at a time. But the fun part is, these thoughts and images can move and adapt. If there's a way to make them darker, scarier, closer to home, then that OCD worm will find a way. It's all-consuming in a way I can't quite explain. There is *nothing* else in your life.

Eventually you adapt or quite literally die. OCD has a higher suicide rate than the general population. It's listed as one of the UN's top ten most debilitating disorders. Somewhere around 12.5 per cent of OCD sufferers will attempt suicide in their lifetime. But that's not because they *want* to die. It's because they just want it to *stop*. When I say sufferers, I mean it in the truest sense of the word. You can't switch your brain off if it's not playing ball. You can't avoid your OCD themes in your sleep – for me they just warped into night terrors where I would be physically kicking and punching, fighting for my life. My husband trying to hold my limbs down so I didn't hurt myself. Simple pleasures like watching nonsense telly or reading a trashy book were a total no-no. You can't concentrate, and at any time the next word on the page might generate a whole new slew of deeply dark, nightmarish brainwaves. So, you do what you can to try and stop or neutralise the thoughts. But that's like trying to hold back the tide or stop the sun from rising. It takes a long time to learn or re-learn that it's not the thoughts themselves that are the problem, it's your *reaction* to them.

I was terrified to google my symptoms in those early months, absolutely convinced that a government SWAT team would crash through my bedroom door and windows at three in the morning because I'd googled 'having scary thoughts about my baby', 'unwanted sexual and violent thoughts, new mum'. Even writing this now, I'm so wary that it may mean having my baby taken away. What kind of a mother, what kind of a person, has disgusting ideas about their tiny baby when bathing or feeding or changing them? The fact that I had even had these thoughts in the first place was proof enough for me that I was obviously, even unbeknownst to me, a monster. I couldn't believe I didn't see it before.

OCD's favourite game is What If? What if I'm bathing my baby and under the fog of utter exhaustion, zone out for a moment and he slips under the water? What if I black out and do something dreadful and then come to, to find I'm holding his tiny head beneath the bathwater? What if I just let it happen?

What if I just sit there doing nothing as my baby fights for breath? Could I do that? Would I do that? And then most terrifying of all, do I want to do that? Judging by my repulsion and agitation at the idea, I didn't *think* so. But thinking so wasn't sure enough.

Changing the baby on the kitchen island, I would be living in two realities. One where, from the outside, a mother is going through the motions of taking off the wet or soiled nappy, cleaning the area and putting on a fresh one. But simultaneously, skewing reality to the left a touch, I would be seeing two to three seconds into the future. And not just seeing, almost feeling and hearing it. I could smell blood that hadn't been spilled. Hear phantom crying. What if I looked away for a moment and he rolled off the changing mat onto our cold, black-tiled kitchen floor? I could hear the crack-splat of his skull hitting the deck. And I would just stand there. Not acting, not knowing what to do. Imagining my husband walking in with a shocked 'what have you done?!?'

The fear of doing something wrong that could never be undone became my sole obsession. Once a baby dies, they're dead. Once you've touched something, it cannot be untouched. Once you've had a thought, it cannot be unthunk. Meanwhile, in the real world, I was finishing up the final poppers on his onesie, picking him back up and moving onto the next task. My elevated heart rate, sometimes 135 bpm according to my smartwatch, would be the only telltale sign that anything had just happened. But for me *everything* had happened and everything had changed. What if I dropped him walking up the stairs, or forgot I was carrying him and just let my arms drop to my sides? I'd be looking over the banister seeing him unmoving in a pool of slowly expanding crimson blood. A crime scene. One I had created. And I could never undo that. You can't undrop something. The laws of physics don't work that way. The police would arrive. Would they believe me? Would I believe me?

The closest explanation to someone who doesn't have OCD and can't understand it is the Airport Feeling. You know when you're going through airport security, and even though you know without a shadow of a doubt that you didn't pack a homemade bomb or twenty kilos of heroin, *just* as your bag is being X-rayed there's suddenly an element of mistrust? You're not a terrorist or a drug mule – you'd have remembered. But *WHAT IF*. What if someone else put them in your bag, or you did pack something illegal while you were distracted or drunk or sleepwalking. You could have accidentally thrown a bread knife in your rucksack along with your passport and charger, too busy running around to notice. You didn't mean to. You probably didn't. But there *is* a possibility. And that's where OCD metastasises. Maybe any minute, you're going to be pulled aside, arrested and have your life ruined.

Your heart rate shows a flicker of elevation but then your luggage sails through and you move on to duty-free, thinking, 'huh, that was weird'. It's that, but over and over. On repeat. You never make it through security. Your bags are put back on the conveyor belt to be checked, checked and checked again. It's a sort of purgatory. Each time, you *know* there's nothing in your bags but each time, there's a moment of hesitancy. Until that uniformed security officer doesn't stand up with a finger pointed, *j'accuse* written all over his grim face, you won't be sure. But even when nothing happens, the relief is short-lived. There *is* no duty-free and departure lounge for you. And so you dutifully head back to the start of the queue waiting to grab your grey plastic tray to be checked again. Ad infinitum.

Yet another fascinating facet of my illness – if this was an illness – was that I wanted to make myself as small as possible. I didn't want to take up any room, physically or metaphorically. I'd stick to two or three small spots in our house. It didn't feel like my home anymore. I was disgusting and sullied everything I touched, and I likely wouldn't be here soon anyway, so symbolically I didn't get too comfortable once I came home from the hospital. Something as simple as going in rooms I'd been avoiding and deciding to add something or move an object, was huge for me. Another permission. I had every right to be there. I didn't have to play the role of this ghostly lodger I'd cast myself in. My husband begged me to make myself more at home – in my own fucking home. God, the brain is wild.

★

Before realising I had OCD, I'd thought it was all neatness and germs. I'm a huge Poirot fan and his watch words were 'order and method'. While Agatha Christie never explicitly wrote that he had obsessive compulsive disorder, there were certainly marked traits. I loved Poirot as a character because he was so different from me. His thoughts were ordered and he always, always pushed through the confusion and red herrings and got to the right answer. Everything and everyone had its place. He was all-knowing; I was all-doubting. On the surface I was a high achiever but underneath, I was a mental flounderer with a foggy brain. I couldn't have OCD. Howard Hughes had OCD. He was a germophobic recluse. Jack Nicholson won an Oscar for his portrayal of an OCD-riddled romance writer characterised by rigid routines and strong superstitions. I wasn't like that. His contamination subtype meant he could only use disposable cutlery and washed his hands excessively or would check and recheck locks and switches. I didn't do any of that. Did I? I was nothing like any of them. Was I?

Then I remembered that when I was pregnant, I'd developed some of the physical checking behaviours that I had never displayed before. I would always go up to bed first, as I liked to read while my husband would stay in the living room to watch some god-awful sci-fi. I would pad along our cold, Victorian tiled hallway to lock the front door. He would always forget, and I had vivid visions of a stranger wandering in off the street, quietly murdering my husband and then coming upstairs to give me and my baby a Sharon Tate-style ending. It wasn't hugely conscious, not like later scenarios would become. I just thought it was probably a natural symptom of pregnancy, becoming more protective of your bump and mitigating dangerous circumstances around yourself to protect that bump. In the blink of an eye, it just meant turning back and making sure I *had* just turned the key like I thought I had. But each time I reached the bottom stair, I wouldn't be convinced with my new baby brain that I had just locked it. Maybe I was remembering doing it last night. I would do this several times going back and forth, but it didn't cause me any considerable distress, so I didn't think too much about it.

The general thesis of OCD is that if you don't do X, you will get Y. A simple premise and one that most people use every day. If you don't buy milk, you don't have milk. If you don't wash your hands, your hands will be dirty. But where OCD-ers deviate is the belief that if you don't do X, a seemingly small task, ritual or thought process, you will get Y, consequences so dire, that really doing this one, trivial little thing over and over and over is a small price to pay. Pathological superstition. You've washed your hands, they are now 'clean'. But what is clean? How clean is clean enough? And in the moments after washing and drying them, have I re-contaminated them? Is this water tainted, has this soap been tampered with, is this towel sanitary, are there germs and bugs I can't see with the naked eye? What if I infect my loved ones or myself with a toxic disease and everyone dies? Not sure? Better start again then. Rinse, then repeat. Pun intended.

OCD thinking is truly ego-dystonic, a posh way of saying the thoughts go against your values and who you are. This thinking is found in all types of OCD, but it is considered that a person's OCD behaviours will fall into one of these five main categories according to OCD UK.[2] (but there can be overlapping between categories too):

Checking
Contamination/Mental Contamination
Symmetry and Ordering
Ruminations/Intrusive Thoughts
Hoarding

However, within these categories lay different subtypes. Your particular flavour of OCD if you will. Remember, OCD attacks what you most value and subtypes can overlap too. Here are just a handful of examples:

Scrupulosity OCD: Imagine a deeply religious person has the intrusive thought that they suddenly just stand up and blaspheme in their place of worship. They don't want to – they're mortified at the very idea and want nothing more than to unthink it – so, they pray. But they don't do it right or 'mean' it sufficiently and so they start again, but it's never quite enough.

Sexual Orientation OCD: A person will innately know their sexuality but obsessively wonder if they're being truthful with themselves and their partner.

Sensorimotor OCD: Obsessively concentrating on the sensation of an automatic bodily function like blinking, breathing and swallowing or whether you're sweating or aroused.

Relationship OCD: The fear and compulsive need to check if you love your partner, the worry that even unbeknownst to you, you may have cheated on them.

Existential OCD: Unrelenting intrusive thoughts about life, death and reality. What if I don't really exist? Do I really have free will?

At points, I daydreamed about having one of these other sub-types of OCD. I'd take anything. Those others didn't bother me as much, so I could just dedicate, say, seventy per cent of my day to that obsession and subsequent compulsions. It'd be fun, finding out what they were. The parameters I confined myself to were so preposterously defined, I could have just wished away OCD altogether. But that would have been silly.

Oh no, I knew I *had* to have OCD but if I could just have the Contamination kind or maybe the Sexual Orientation subset, things would be easier. Those didn't worry me nearly as much. I'd promise to commit a good amount of my life to the altar of obsessive compulsive disorder but maybe I could be a vicar rather than a priest and then have some semblance of a normal life around it? Not go the whole hog. But it felt like this unholy church would accept nothing less than total obedience and devotion.

The sub-types I struggled with were Sensorimotor OCD (constantly checking and tuning into my heartbeat or groinal area), Counting OCD (not tolerating anything outside of a multiple of five, silently counting to myself during every task or giving myself arbitrary countdowns: for example, I *must* get to the baby within ten seconds of him crying or he might die), Real Event OCD (taking a seemingly small, insignificant moment and replaying it over and over to check nothing 'bad' happened). But by far the worst, most disturbing and truly soul-destroying, the real elephant in the room, was Paedophile Obsessive Compulsive Disorder. For obvious reasons, this is one of the most taboo and hardest to talk about sub-types of OCD, and subsequently one of the least reported. My skin is prickling and I'm getting 'hot neck' just writing this. I've never explained or discussed it in these blatant terms, so stick with me while I figure it out as I go.

For some context, years earlier, my husband and I had been in Los Angeles. I had been having meetings and auditions, and we'd fitted in a little holiday. LA is an incredible place, unlike anywhere I'd ever known before. Certainly, different from auditioning in London, where things were a little more conservative and had more gravity. Hollywood was all loud and open and when you asked someone how they were, they actually told you. There was no tight-lipped, polite, British, 'I'm fine, thank you, how are you?' It was more: 'Well, I'm good today actually, I had a great session with my therapist yesterday and I'm working through my feelings of self-worth. So, what did you think of the script?'

While there, we were invited to the premiere of *Precious* at Mann's famous Chinese Theatre on Hollywood Boulevard and were enchanted by the celebrity handprints in the cement leading up to this historic cinema. My husband was thrilled to find an impression of John Wayne's fist. We still have a photo of him grinning up at the camera, his fist nestled into the impression that once housed the Hollywood great.

We found the red carpet, eyes peeled for famous actors. We saw Verne Troyer. This was it. From being a nobody girl from a small Welsh village to being in Hollywood and witnessing Mariah Carey being led out on stage by two, what I can only describe as, heel handlers (her stilettos were so sky high, she required two muscled hunks to help her put one foot in front of the other) felt incredible. Surreal but incredible. There was Oscar buzz around the film, especially for Mariah, as she hadn't worn any make-up for the character and her hair was a mousy brown, simply tied back in a bobble. So brave. Almost like a normal person.

Harvey Weinstein was a couple of rows ahead of us with two younger, very beautiful women, one on either side of him, but this was 2009 and we didn't know about all that yet. We got free popcorn which, in America, you pour melted butter over. Mind-blowing cultural difference there. We were a couple of Luddites continually playing with the butter-tap, not believing what we were seeing. And so we all settled to watch the film. The story of *Precious* is pretty harrowing. Set in 1980s Harlem, Claireece 'Precious' Jones lives with her sexually violent and verbally abusive single mother. Her now-absent father raped her, resulting in two pregnancies, the first baby being born with Down's Syndrome. The second baby was born under her mother's ire, as she's intensely jealous that her husband desired their daughter over his own wife. Precious must have tempted him away somehow. Her hatred is visceral. Her father dies from AIDs and Precious will discover she is HIV-positive, too.

It's uncompromisingly miserable and by the end when everyone's clapping, I was a sobbing wreck. My husband dismissed it as misery porn. We'd been invited to the after-party with Mariah freaking Carey but I was in no state to go, so we headed back to the cheap apartment we'd been renting. As soon as we got there, I realised I'd dropped my passport inside the theatre, so my poor husband had to go back and convince security to let him back in. Total disaster of an evening, but why do I mention it? There's a moment in *Precious* where the title character says the sexual abuse with her mother and father began while she was a baby, lying in between them in bed. Why am I telling you this? Because that moment in the film was all I could think about after having the baby. It haunted me. It tortured me. What if I fell asleep next to him and did something terrible and couldn't remember? It consumed every part of me.

★

Imagine you're naturally a very protective person, especially over vulnerable things: children or animals, for example. It's in your nature to be on edge on their behalf when the need arises. A lot of people feel this empathy, it's part of human nature, but some feel it more than others. Where OCD-ers veer off into the extreme, here is the need to ask the question 'why?'. 'Why do I feel so defensive over things that can't protect themselves as well as I can? Is it a genuine intention to safeguard or is it something more disturbing?' If OCD can question whether something is sinister, then it will go to town. It could be anything, I promise. For example, I just looked up and saw an apple. Surely, it's hard to have sinister thoughts about a nice, crunchy Pink Lady? Well, buckle up and watch – you're about to see OCD do its thing.

When I see an apple, I might think about the poisoned apple from the Snow White fairytale. My son's absolute favourite fruit is an apple; he gets through a bushel a week. What if he chokes on a lump of apple flesh? What if I accidentally gave him a contaminated one? What if something went wrong in the supply chain and it's chock full of a dangerous level of pesticide? The supermarket will have to 'recall' it, there'll be a class action suit: the Snow White Generation inadvertently poisoned by apples. Or what if someone out there has laced apples with a narcotic and dotted them throughout local fruit aisles à la the 1980s Tylenol Murders? When I was little, I heard that apple pips contain cyanide. (They actually contain amygdalin, which releases trace amounts of cyanide when chewed or broken down and you would literally need to eat hundreds in one sitting for it to have the *slightest* effect.) I also worried when I was very young that if I accidentally swallowed an apple seed, a huge apple tree would grow out of my belly, Jack and the Beanstalk-style. What if that happens to my baby?

As I've mentioned, I love Agatha Christie's books. In the Poirot novels, the character Ariadne Oliver, a mystery writer, is loosely based on Christie herself. Her motif is that she is always munching on apples, can't get enough of them, until, in *Hallowe'en Party* (1969), a young girl is found drowned in a galvanised steel bucket of bobbing apples in front of the fireplace during . . . well, a Halloween party. Ariadne Oliver vows to never eat another apple again.

This sounds like I've really thought about it and that I deliberately chose the example of an apple as it has so much symbolism, but believe me, I genuinely just looked up, saw an apple and started typing. So, let's think where else we could go? Oh, I know – the film *American Pie*, shagging an apple pie? You could have sex with an apple. Not sure how that would work for a woman or for a man, now I think about it (drill a hole, I guess) but it's put some funky images in your head, hasn't it? Or, don't two apples look a bit like two boobs? My point is that if I can run away on just one simple thought about a fruit I'm not particularly attached to, then what happens when it comes to something I regard as utterly precious and vulnerable and would never, ever want to hurt?

That's how easily a person with OCD can jump from feeling like something needs to be protected and treasured to thinking that they might unknowingly be a danger to it. Am I a secret child abuser with ulterior motives towards children or am I feeling a natural, maternal instinct? He's so cute, I really want to hold him. But why? What's the motive? Don't most normal people just 'know' that they're not a danger and move on with their day? Is the fact I'm even questioning it proof enough that I'm a predator? I haven't ever hurt a child before or even wanted to, the complete opposite actually; my only focus is on keeping everyone safe, but it only takes one thought, one moment, for all that to change. Maybe I'm one of those nice child abusers who doesn't want to abuse children? Even writing this is making my OCD spike and claw at me to investigate.

But there is nothing to investigate. If you desperately want to protect your precious tiny baby from every conceivable harm, then what could be better for your OCD mind to conjure up than all the ways in which you are the thing you most fear? Then add a good splash of sleep deprivation, a healthy dollop of hormonal chaos and this thing has legs. Then finally attach the societal hysteria around anything to do with the subject – every time I switched on the news or a new TV show, it was all about child abuse or abductions or death – and now you can't tell anyone about your worries because they won't understand or they'll report you or they'll never really look at you the same way again. Will they always wonder if any of this could be true, too?

From my experience, the answer is unequivocally no.

The problem with spotting that I had OCD lay in the fact that almost all my compulsions were in my mind. I didn't present as physically as other sufferers, so unless I was very honest about what was going on up there, I was going to get left behind. They reckon it can take between ten and fifteen years from the onset of OCD symptoms to a diagnosis. According to that, I was bang on track. It seemed that unless you're showing the outside world what it thinks it needs to see, then you're looked over for the correct diagnosis and there are two main problems with this. Firstly and most cruelly of all, OCD can often be misdiagnosed as general anxiety disorder or depression, as it was for me, and while these conditions can go hand in hand with OCD (I mean, who the hell wouldn't be anxious or depressed if they couldn't be around a knife and their baby at the same time, because your terrified, sleep-deprived, hormone-riddled mind can only absorb the simple equation that knife plus baby could equal dead baby).

Secondly, OCD gaslights you into believing that you don't have the disorder at all. And how do you know that's not true? It's a hall of mirrors where you can't even tell what's the *real* you and what's simply a distorted reflection. Soon the reflections outnumber you and then you start to doubt you're even at a fairground attraction at all. You frantically search for a fire-exit sign but it's just more mirrors. You're stuck and everywhere you turn, there are more echoes of another, darker you. Mirrors within mirrors. Running around helplessly looking for a way out but moving deeper into the twisted, refracted reality. But the thing about a mirror is that it's not a true representation of you to begin with. When you look at your face in the mirror, you're already at a disadvantage because it's a flipped image. Your face doesn't actually look like that. And the smallest thing can affect the image your brain transmits back. The light, the angle, cracks, warped glass, compromised vision . . . There are so many variables that misrepresent your true likeness and when those variables are made of intangible puffs of smoke in your mind, you're onto a loser. OCD really is all smoke and mirrors.

INTRUSIVE THOUGHTS

If there were the Ten Commandments of OCD, they would read a little like this:

1. Thou art a monster, perchance?

2. Art thou sure?

3. What if . . . (insert thy variable hither)?

4. Thou shall check once more.

5. Didst thou check properly?

6. Thou shoulds't check again.

7. Thou shall covet another subset.

8. I might not but keep everyone safe.

9. Thou shall journey in vicious circles.

10. Thou canst not say to anyone lest thou be cast out.

It took me such a long time to see and know that what I was doing was constant risk-assessing. I was hypervigilant, not thinking as rationally as I should, and the idea of any harm coming to my baby scared me right down to the very core of my being. So, knife plus baby could easily equal dead baby when that was the outcome I was trying to avoid most of all. I know that some women will refuse to go in the kitchen, throw out all sharp objects, ask their partners to prepare food – anything to stop the possibility of harm coming to the baby. This is really doing a compulsion by proxy. Told you OCD was a tricky fucker. And when you run out of all the ways something could accidentally occur, the only variable left that you can't control is your own mind. As evidenced by having these horrid thoughts, intrusive images and false urges in the first place. It's a macabre carousel. It always reminds me of that line in 'Hotel California' –'you can check out any time you like but you can never leave'. Until that awful moment, three months in, when I'd responded adversely to a change in medication, and I realised there was a way to make this stop. That I could, indeed, check out.

★

Confiding in a person of authority about what was happening to me was the biggest leap of faith I have ever taken. From there, I had a mixture of responses: some incredibly insightful, others disastrous and a couple, and I don't say this lightly, nearly fatal.

I couldn't understand what had happened and was still happening to me. I'd never heard of a new mother unable to turn her thoughts off. It was a 24/7 merry-go-round and no matter how sick or disorientated I became, the revolting roundabout kept on turning. I just needed a minute, to press pause on this descent into matrescence – a word I wouldn't hear for years to come. The term matrescence was coined by anthropologist Dana Raphael as 'the process of becoming a mother'. Likened to puberty, it's the hormonal, physical, emotional and social transition into motherhood and I would bet my last quid that the Perinatal Mental Health Service I was assigned to still haven't heard of it.

Matrescence took over every area of my life. Physically, I almost couldn't bear the changes. I've often described intense OCD as wearing someone else's skin and that applies here too. It wasn't mine, it didn't fit, it didn't feel like me, it was uncomfortable, and I just wanted to peel it off like a grotesque wetsuit. Leave it in a festering puddle on the floor and scrub myself clean. But I couldn't, and I didn't understand any of it and so,

INTRUSIVE THOUGHTS

justifiably and perfectly normally, I decided I had been cursed. No one changes overnight like this. But if I heard someone say 'you're not the first woman to give birth' one more time, I was very likely to scream. I get it, okay? I get that millions of women have done this all over the world for more than two hundred millennia and I'm the only one to get it so catastrophically wrong. Thank you for the reminder. I wish more than anyone that I could be that paragon of Woman who gives birth using nothing but my own breath and drinks a nutritional smoothie made of my own placenta. But I'm not, okay? I'm this. This . . . fiasco of a female. Fuck.

Apparently, now I was the kind of woman who cried when her baby did that rooting thing with his little mouth. I was the girl huddled in an armchair while her husband held their baby on the other side of the room, watching them like a haunted owl. I was the woman who trembled while putting new Milton tablets in the steriliser. You didn't have to tell me I was fucked up – I knew that. What I didn't know was why and how to fix it. I was pleading with Perinatal Mental Health to furnish me with answers, but I was misunderstood, not listened to, or fobbed off with the promise of leaflets that would arrive in the post in six weeks' time. Let's hope I wasn't dead by then. Though the tribunal would have served them right.

At the end of one harrowing week, my husband insisted we got some fresh air. It'd be good for us. It was nearing 5pm on a Friday afternoon. We parked, set up the unnecessarily complicated pram and set off on our crisp, autumnal walk. My phone rang and my heart sank. It read PNMH (Perinatal Mental Health) – I'd been expecting to hear from them days ago. I told the nurse on the phone that nothing had changed; in fact, things were getting darker. She didn't seem bothered. She asked me if I was having any suicidal ideation, I replied truthfully that I was. She proceeded to ask if I 'planned on doing anything this weekend?' I told her no; I couldn't do that to my husband. I obviously gave the right answer as she signed off for the weekend with the promise of yet more leaflets that would take weeks to arrive. My husband tried to gauge how the phone call had gone; I shook my head sadly, overcome with despair. Still, a nice walk would do me good. It didn't.

I was in constant contact with PNMH – if you can call somebody promising to call me back immediately and hearing from a completely different person with no knowledge of my case about a week later, constant. There's a form they ask you to answer in the immediate postpartum period called the Edinburgh Postnatal Depression Scale (EPDS) and it seemed to me that they would keep asking me until I scored sufficiently low enough to get me off the books. It's a really fun, ten-item, get-to-know-you quiz.

EDINBURGH POSTNATAL DEPRESSION SCALE[3]

Please select the answer that comes closest to how you have felt in the past 7 days:

1. I have been able to laugh and see the funny side of things

As much as I always could
Not quite so much now
Definitely not so much now
Not at all

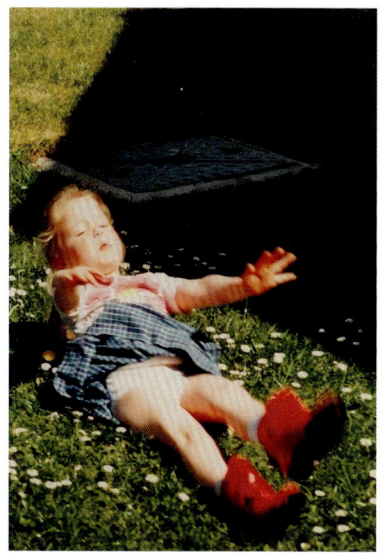
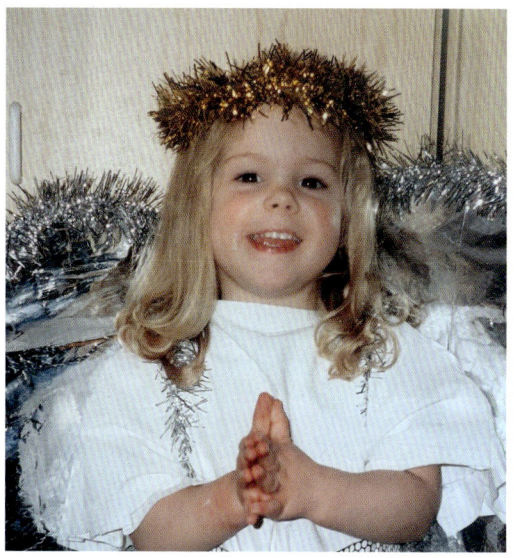

Graceful since 1985.

I can feel her tiny brain fizzing from here. I want to reach back and hug her, tell her it will all be okay.

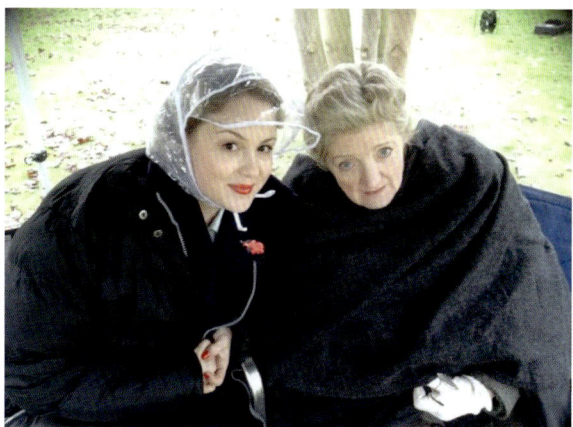

Reunited with Julia Mackenzie on the set of *Marple* in December 2012. We worked together on my first ever job, *Cranford*.

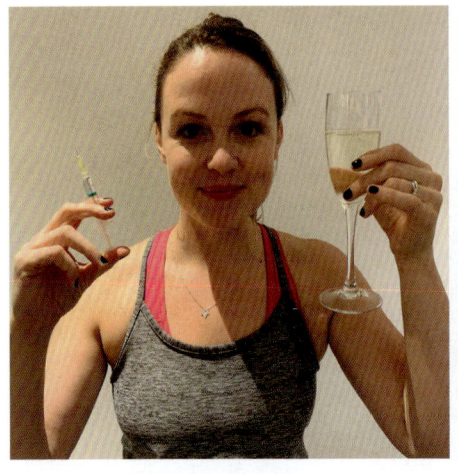

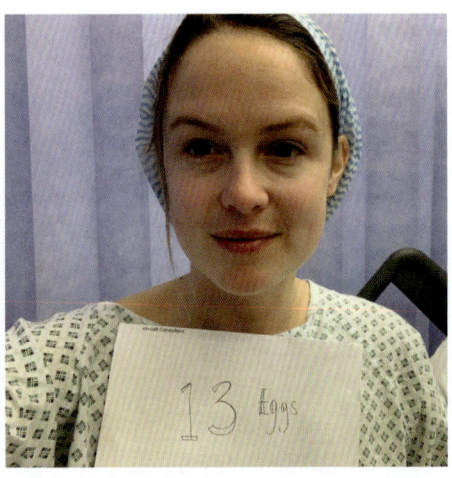

First jab for IVF, post Zumba with a glass of fizz. The most middle-class photo of my life.

Bumper crop! Thirteen eggs.

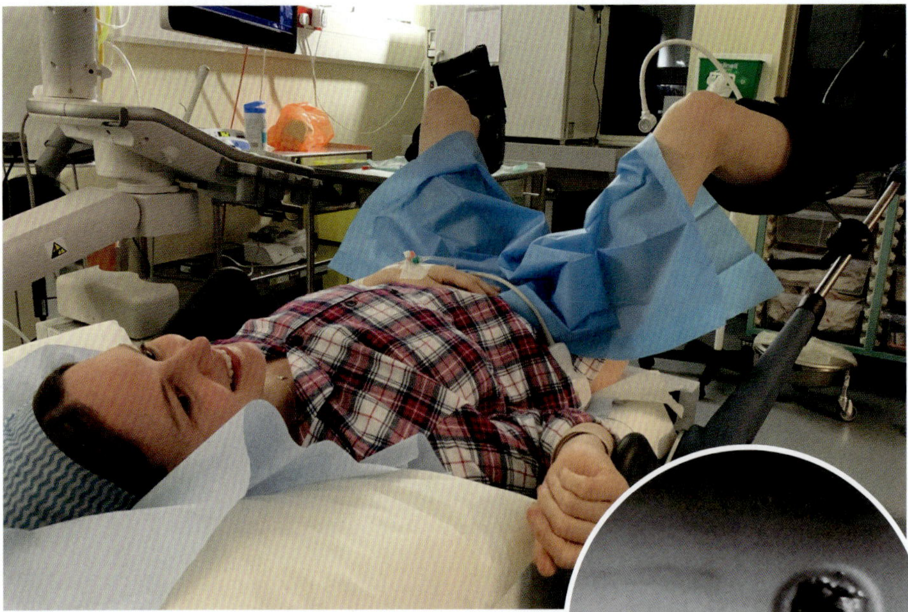

Missed my cue. Removing my knickers for the embryo transfer.

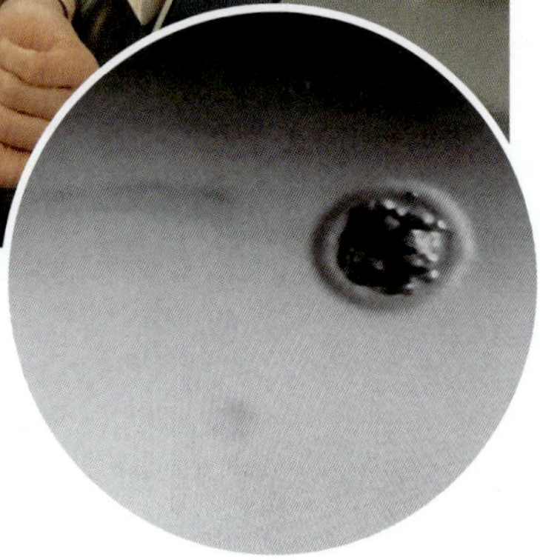

Our beautifully collapsed third embryo aka our son.

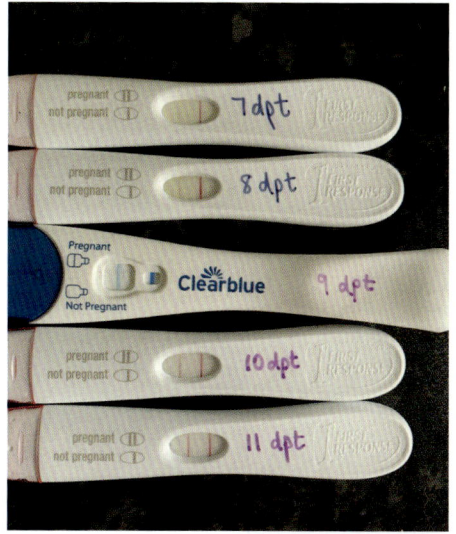
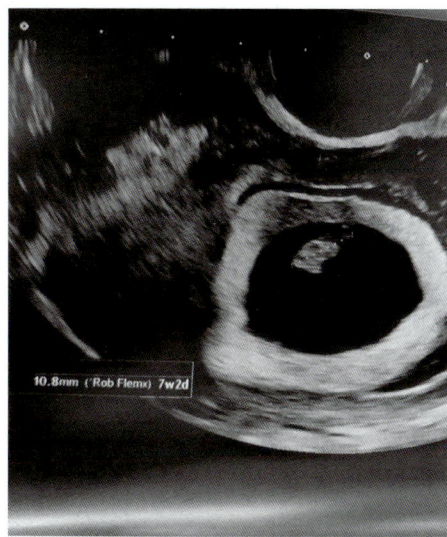
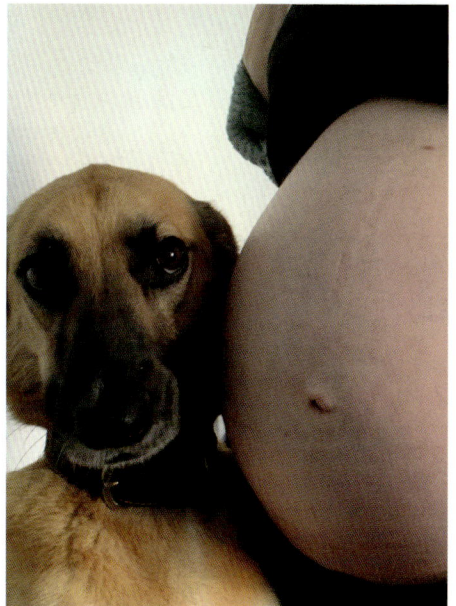
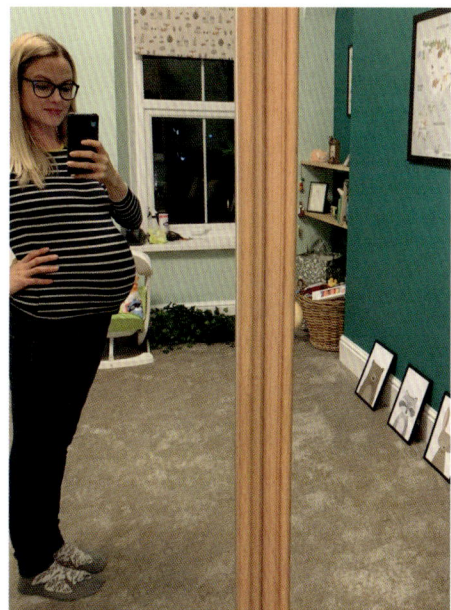

Top left: Illicit testing, flouting the Two-Week Wait rule. (DPT means Days Post-Transfer).

Top right: The emergency early pregnancy scan that revealed our little guy still had a heartbeat.

Bottom left: Bob and bump.

Bottom right: Feeling like I'm in my own rom-com montage. Decorating the nursery and blooming pregnancy. It's all coming together.

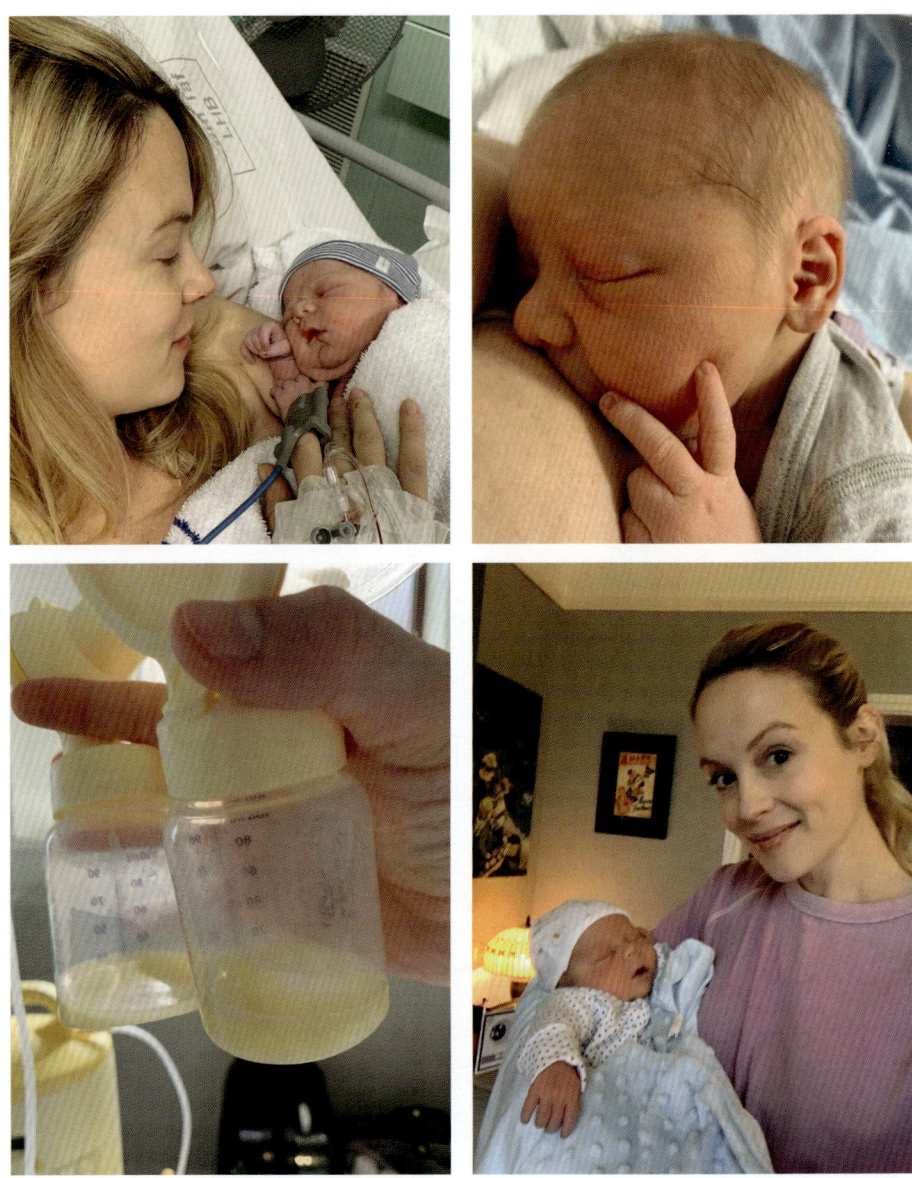

Top left: He's here! I feel weird – hooked up to two blood transfusions. Not long after my husband took this photograph, my son would be whisked away from me.

Top right: Breastfeeding is excruciating. But I like that he has some attitude already.

Bottom left: Hard-won colostrum quarry.

Bottom right: This is the selfie I took to post on my private Facebook page, for friends and family to see. While I looked fine, I was becoming really unwell and burst into tears straight after the photo was taken.

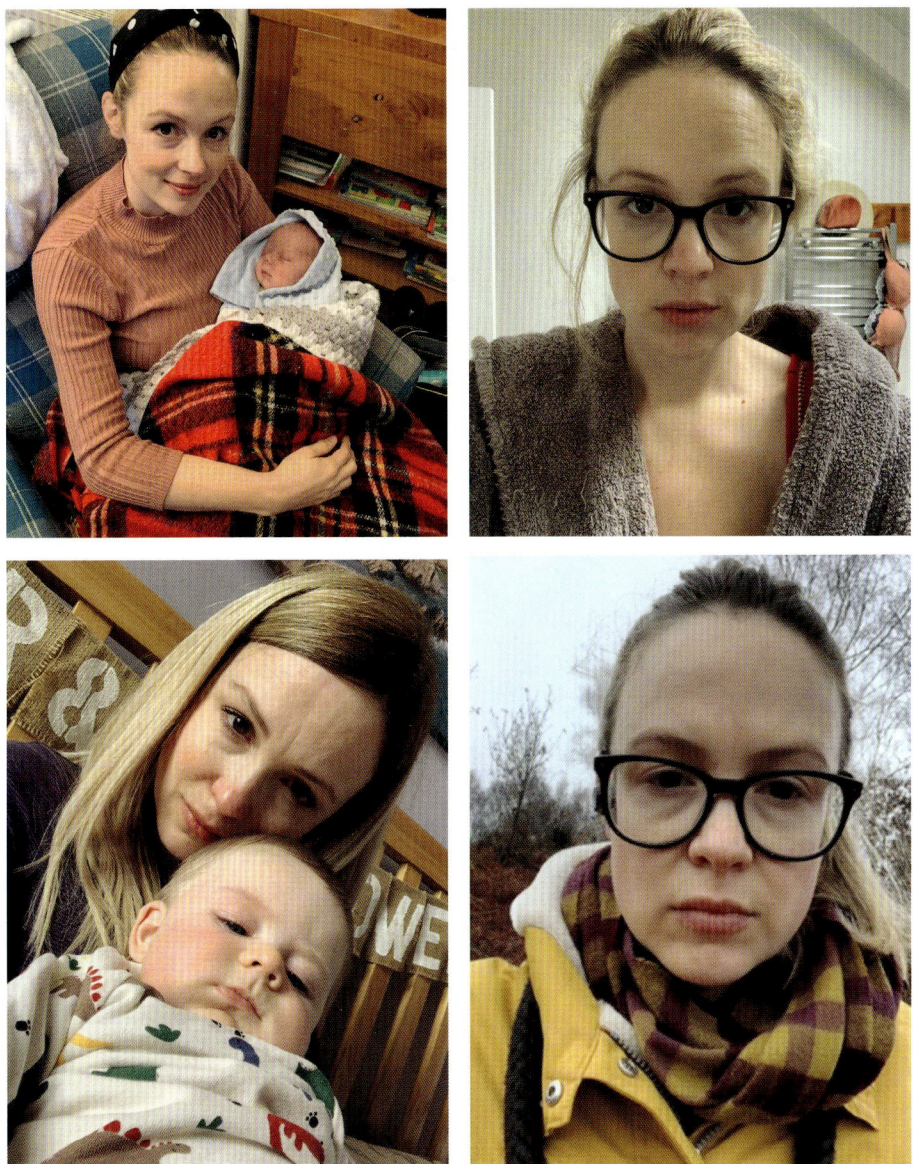

Top left: Not eating, not sleeping; OCD has its hooks in me. But all I'm told is that I look 'amazing' and how lucky I am to have 'lost the baby weight so fast'.

Top right: Two weeks postpartum and I'm shrinking away.

Bottom left: Why can't I do this like everyone else? He's so perfect. I just want to be a good mam to him.

Bottom right: 27th January 2021. I stop myself in my tracks while walking the dog, knowing I have a way out. I take this picture hoping my husband will see it later and just understand.

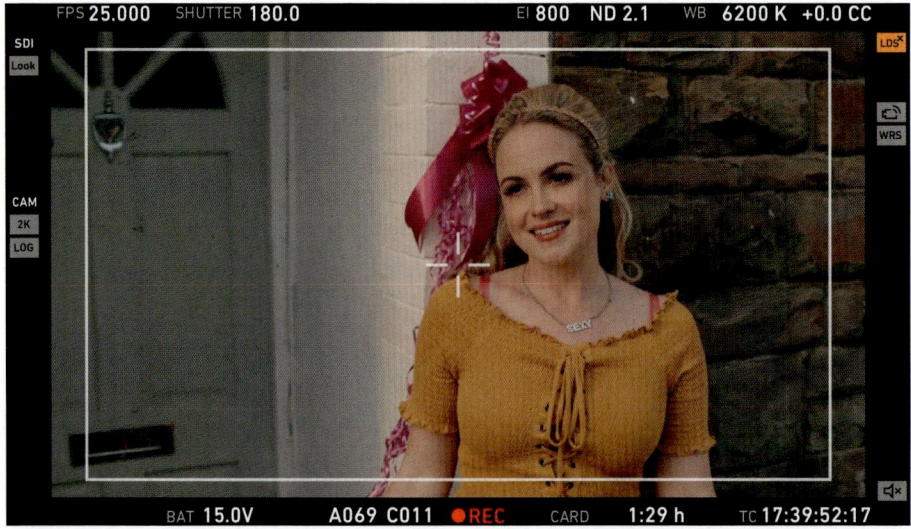

On the set of *The Tuckers*, ten months postpartum. Full make-up, full smiles, masking a miserable existence. You can't always tell.

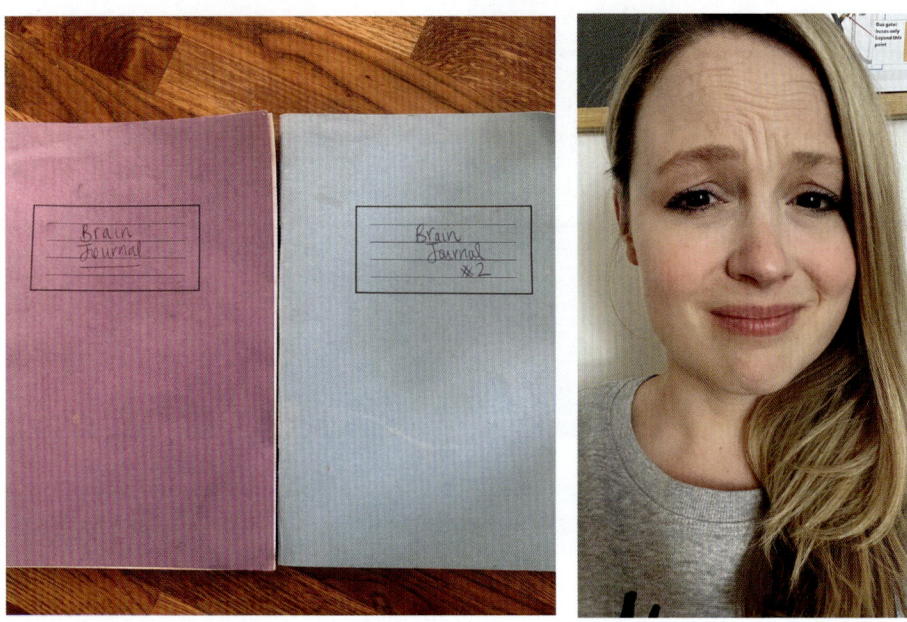

Left: My brain journals.

Right: In the waiting room, just before an ERP session.

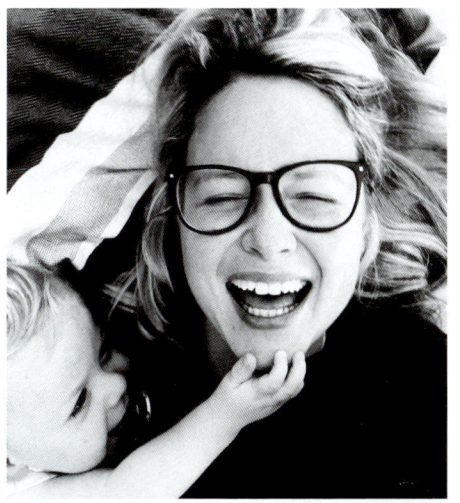
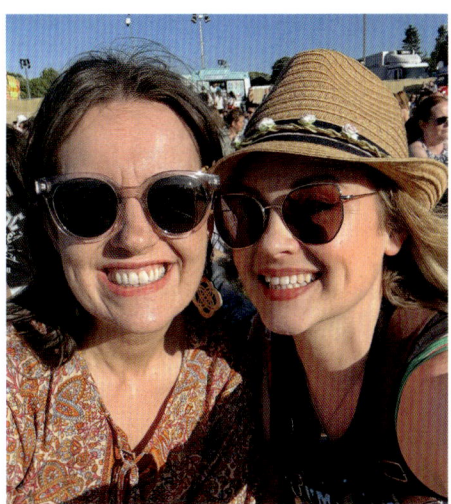
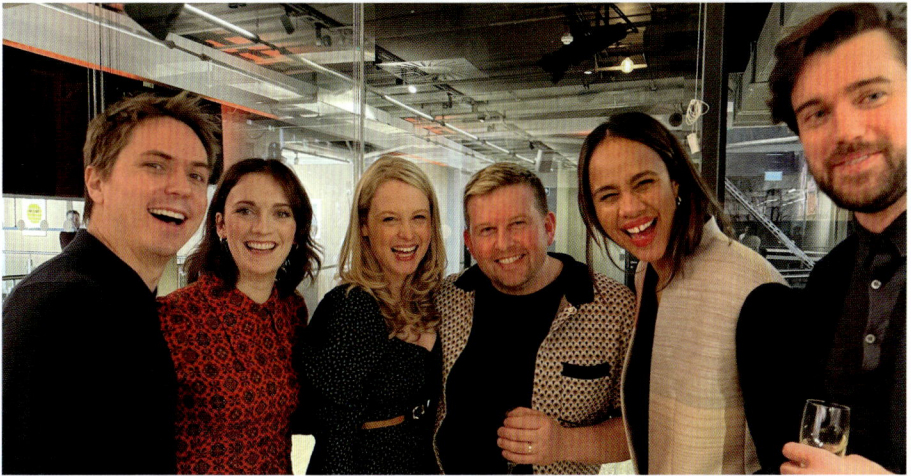
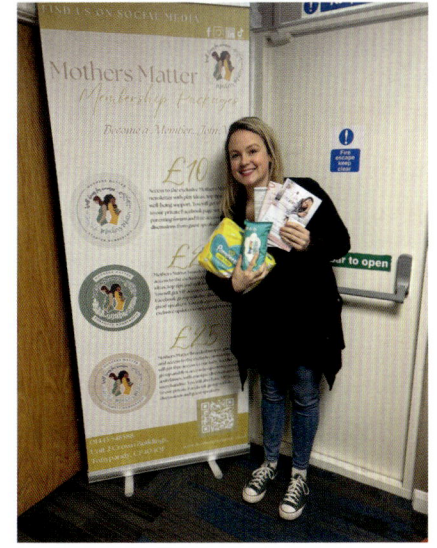

Top left: Learning it's okay to smile, laugh and enjoy being a mam to my little boy.

Top right: Jess and I have been friends since we were eleven. Here we are reliving our youth at the Alanis Morissette concert in Cardiff in July 2025.

Above: *Fresh Meat* ten-year reunion at the BFI, London.

Right: At Mothers Matter in Tonypandy, where I learned there were other women like me. I am now a proud patron of the charity.

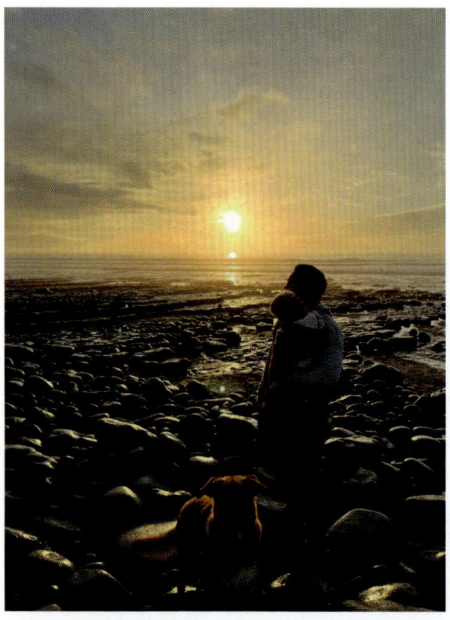

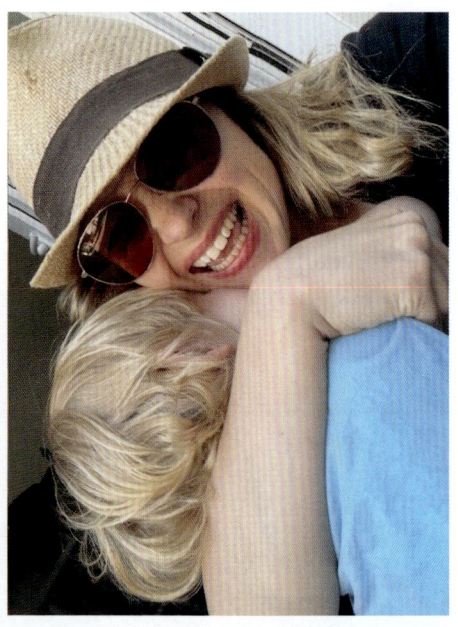

The day I squatted in a freezing rock pool at Southerndown beach.

Laughing with my beautiful boy. We have the most wonderful bond.

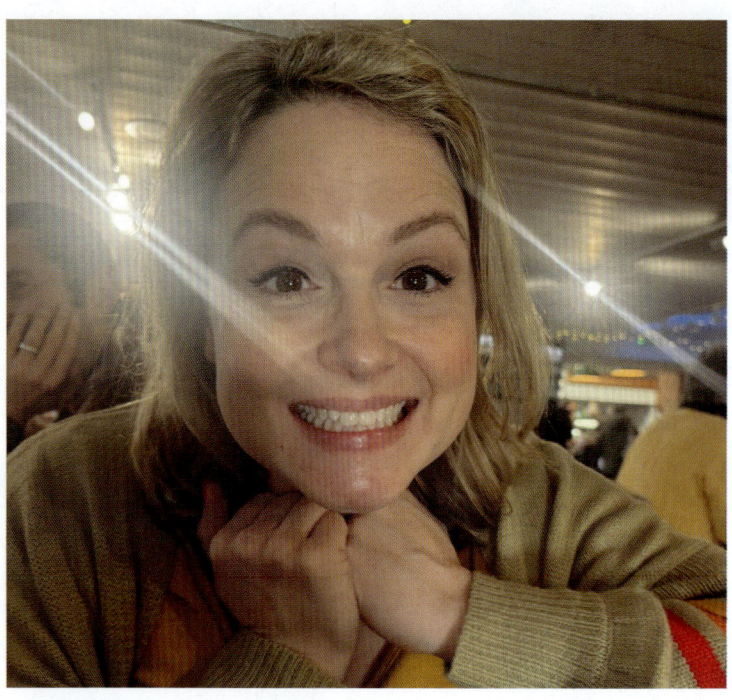

A photo my 5-year-old son took of me. Amazing to see myself through his eyes.

INTRUSIVE THOUGHTS

2. I have looked forward with enjoyment to things

As much as I ever did
Rather less than I used to
Definitely less than I used to
Hardly at all

3. I have blamed myself unnecessarily when things went wrong

Yes, most of the time
Yes, some of the time
Not very often
No, never

4. I have been anxious or worried for no good reason

No, not at all
Hardly ever
Yes, sometimes
Yes, very often

5. I have felt scared or panicky for no good reason

Yes, quite a lot
Yes, sometimes
No, not much
No, not at all

6. Things have been getting on top of me

Yes, most of the time I haven't been able to cope at all
Yes, sometimes I haven't been coping as well as usual
No, most of the time I have coped quite well
No, I have been coping as well as ever

7. I have been so unhappy that I have had difficulty sleeping

Yes, most of the time
Yes, sometimes
Not very often
No, not at all

8. I have felt sad or miserable

Yes, most of the time
Yes, quite often
Not very often
No, not at all

9. I have been so unhappy that I have been crying

Yes, most of the time
Yes, quite often
Only occasionally
No, never

10. The thought of harming myself has occurred to me

Yes, quite often
Sometimes
Hardly ever
Never

INTRUSIVE THOUGHTS

Ten questions, three points an answer. I consistently scored 30/30 on this scale. If you score more than 10, it's advised they look further into it. For months, a different person would ask me these questions on the phone and my heart would break as I answered as honestly as I could, as I knew that's what it would take to get better. I was told early on that appointments with the perinatal psychiatrist were 'gold dust' and I didn't qualify.

Until, eventually, I did.

On a dog walk somewhere in the woods, a nurse called to ask if I had time to go through a thorough record of everything that had happened. I sobbed against a tree as I told her everything, from crashing after the birth, the trauma of the hospital to having unrelenting, unwanted thoughts of harm around my baby for months on end. And I just had to trust that she wouldn't call the police or take my baby from me. She was lovely. So sympathetic and understanding, and she was one of the first people to reassure me that new mums get intrusive thoughts. We spoke for forty minutes. She took it all down and explained it would all be passed on to the doctor. I would only have a forty-five-minute phone appointment, and they didn't want me to waste a single precious second of it, so on the day, the psychiatrist would be fully up to speed on my case. I ambled home, broken but hopeful, and prayed I'd be able to hang on for the next few weeks until my appointment. I did continue to decline but I had this lifeline coming my way, if I could hang on by my bleeding, bitten fingernails. This was going to be the turning point. It just had to be.

The day and hour rolled around and, with the baby napping and my husband and I on opposite couches in the living room, we waited. My phone lit up with an Unknown Number.

This was bloody well it. I'd asked my husband to listen in, as I was deliriously tired and emotionally bashed by this point and I didn't want to allow any room for me to misconstrue what I was being told. I needed someone with a clear head to retain the information for me. With a shaky breath, I swiped to answer.

'Hello?' My voice was small and guarded.

'Hello, is this Kimberley?' a male voice asked.

'Yes,' I shuddered out.

'OK, this is Dr So-and So. Can you tell me what the problem is?'

Huh? What did he mean tell him what the problem was? I'd spewed my guts out to another stranger I couldn't see on the phone a few weeks before so we could get right to the heart of the matter in this magical, gold-encrusted appointment.

'I've been feeling really unwell. Very dark, not like myself at all. Having terrible thoughts that I can't get out of my mind.'

'Hmm. Okay. And how pregnant are you?'

I stared at my husband, aghast. He nodded towards the phone for me to trust the process and carry on.

'My son is four months old.'

'Oh, you've already had the baby. Okay. Tell me about these thoughts.'

I steeled myself and couldn't believe that, for what felt like the twentieth time, I was recounting the worst time of my life and revealing the deepest, darkest corners of my soul to yet another stranger. I précised it as best I could. A lowlights reel, if you will.

'Right, okay.'

Was he bored? He sounded bored. My husband rubbed my

hand. He was silently telling me this would all be okay but I could see the doubt in his eyes.

'Firstly, can I just ask if your baby is safe with you?'

WHAT?!? I had been assured that this doctor would be fully aware of my hugely common symptoms and that it was great that I'd asked for help and no one – NOBODY – considered me, in any way, to be a risk. I could barely get through an appointment with my midwife, my health visitor, my practice nurse, my GP, my perinatal mental health nurses, without falling to pieces because I loved my baby so much, I just wanted to get better and figure out why this was happening. I'd cut my own arm off with a rusty saw before I hurt my baby. That's what this whole thing was about!!

My eyes shifted from the phone to my husband, and I mouthed, 'I can't . . .' All trust was gone. He didn't get it. He was supposed to get it. There are four main perinatal mental health conditions: depression, anxiety, OCD and psychosis. And I say perinatal because they can occur during pregnancy as well as after. This was the top guy, *the* perinatal psychiatrist for my health board, and he seemed to have no idea what I was describing. Oh my god, I truly was unfixable. A monster with no chance of redemption. I was ready to end the call but I was terrified to, in case he reported me for not co-operating. Government SWAT team again.

Turned out I was right to hang on the line and hear him out. He went on to give me the most bizarre and bewildering advice I have ever received. He told me that after chatting for a couple of minutes he could tell I was a nice person but had no self-esteem. He told me he wanted me to do something for him. Okay. Here it was – THE magic words that would end this living hell and allow me to enjoy my life again. To love and cherish my baby like I wanted to without this cruel doubt and these pathological compulsions that had fully taken over my life.

Lay it on me, Doc.

'Bake a cake.'

Yep, I'd flipped. I was through the looking-glass, and I was genuinely beginning to hear things now. Maybe it was psychosis, but they'd ruled that out, surely. But maybe I was delusional. That would be nice. It would explain so much. The 24-hour Clockwork Orange, eyes pried open, nightmare cum alternate reality I'd been watching, almost hearing, for months. I mean, it wasn't the outcome I'd wanted but at least it was a fucking scientific explanation. But as I looked back at my husband, his eyes had widened in disbelief. Did he hear it too? Ah, shit. Can't be delusional then. The psychiatrist continued that he would like me to make a cake, bake it, eat it and then tell myself that it was a good cake. Then he'd like me to – yeah, unbelievably he wasn't finished – go to the library (do I have a library card anymore?) and take out a self-help book and – this next bit was very important – *don't* read it all in one go. That would be too much. That would overwhelm me. Read it in small chunks. Was he taking the piss? Overwhelm me? We'd passed *overwhelmed* a long time ago. Overwhelm was a comforting swamp I wish I could go back to. I was in the endgame now.

You know that bit in *Gavin and Stacey*, where Mick is supposed to appear on the evening news and they tell everyone they know, so every acquaintance will be watching that night but then his interview is cut short, and Pam angrily screams 'IS. THAT. IT?' as they gather round the telly? Imagine that but with more milk stains and snotty tears. I silently laughed. My husband didn't know what to say. Flummoxed is probably the best way to describe his face but I also saw the penny begin to drop for him as this golden lifeline turned to dust before our very eyes. What did we do now?

I told the doctor that there was another lockdown and libraries were all closed, and you couldn't buy flour because the whole fucking nation had decided to take up baking banana bread. I told him I couldn't sleep. I was desperate for sleep. He prescribed me some sleeping pills and said goodbye. The whole thing took less than eleven minutes. When the line went dead, my husband muttered, 'I can't believe that just happened.' I later asked him if he hadn't been there to hear it himself, would he have believed my retelling of it later?

'Honestly, no. I don't think I would.'

What do you do in stormy, shark-infested waters when someone's just popped your lifeboat? Hell if I know. What's that? The baby's awake. Back to it. That was it, then. We'd just exhausted every option. I smiled sadly as I stood and said, 'It's okay, I'll get him.' I walked out of the room filled with a sadness so intense, I somehow knew I'd never again be who I once was.

It was interesting how differently we reacted to my NHS treatment so far. My husband was angry on my behalf. Angry and disappointed. He'd watched me answer every awkward question, sob through my story to countless healthcare professionals who I never saw or heard from again, jumped through every hoop and felt I'd been treated very poorly. My GP agreed and made an informal complaint to PNMH on my behalf. The very next day, someone from the service called and asked if it was okay if they popped round. That was odd, considering I'd never had a face-to-face with anyone from PNMH due to Covid. A perinatal bigwig came round, masked up, and asked how my psychiatric appointment had gone the day before. We told her. She just blinked. After making small talk she left bemused and we never heard from her or the psychiatrist again.

My reaction was defeated confirmation. Of course. I was beyond help, just as I'd assumed. A trained authority figure had not been able to recognise my symptoms as something medical and treatable so it must be a personality flaw, which was what I'd feared all along. That was it then. No cure. No hope. I fell further into the whirlpool of intrusive thoughts, and it was lights out. Kimberley had left the building. From that moment on, I was a husk. I went through the daily motions of caring for my son and secretly decided that I'd try my very best to get him to his first birthday before I would just disappear.

My husband found a therapist for me online. She was based in Cardiff, which is only a twenty-five-minute drive from us but that made no difference as the sessions had to be via Zoom – Covid, again. I was lost to my own world in a ball on our tan leather couch; I heard my husband in the background explaining my situation and making me an appointment. Something flickered – would this be the thing? The change in luck, in circumstance, in hope? I heard him ask if she'd ever dealt with postnatal OCD. He smiled over at me and nodded. We started having sessions a few days a week. I was honest again, ever hopeful, but I was by now struggling to believe this would help. She was a nice lady; she helped me to make sense of why I was thinking and feeling the way I was but that didn't make it stop. She was understanding and non-judgemental, but I still didn't get the sense from any clinical professional that they truly 'got it'. It was also £100 a pop and with not really earning in the pandemic and our coffers dwindling by the day with mortgage payments, bills, the cost of having a new baby and now trying to fix my brain, soon money would become a problem.

*

That was the status quo for months. Baby routines, therapy on Zoom with a considerate stranger and the ever-present drowning sensation that I was the lowest of the low, and my symptoms weren't really symptoms at all but monstrous parts of my truest personality. I weirdly got into bird watching. I went to my in-laws — basically my second parents — and they made a fuss over the baby while I sat in a chair by the window and counted different species of bird as part of an RSPB survey they'd had through the post. For a moment, I felt like one of those First World War soldiers convalescing with shellshock at a country estate. Nice blanket over the knees but lost to another world. Another version of me would have scoffed at that. I didn't. I spotted another goldfinch and duly marked it down.

I had another phone call with PNMH, but I'd checked out. At this point I think every interaction with them was making me worse, not better. They did the sodding Edinburgh scale again. I was generally scoring 27 out of 30 but that was only because I could answer the sleep question in the affirmative due to the sleeping pills. She sighed and said there wasn't much else they could do for me. Was I still suicidal? Yeah. Would I act on it? Don't think so.

'Am I okay to release you from our service?'

'Sure.'

We hung up and I laughed humourlessly. I already felt a little freer.

6

Dear Diary

(Or Think Twice – Another Day in Paradise)

When they diagnose you with generalised anxiety disorder or depression, you're whacked on antidepressants and offered cognitive behavioural therapy. CBT is the standard for a lot of mental health conditions but the paradox with OCD is that CBT can make you worse. A kindly therapist asking you 'so, why do you think you're having these thoughts?' is the absolute worst thing you can do with someone like me, in the throes of a full-blown OCD episode.

My CBT therapist was a private therapist, paid for out of my actress nest egg, which I'd been squirrelling away for years ready for a rainy, unemployed day. I was also offered six weeks of group Zoom therapy on the NHS in six weeks' time. I couldn't wait that long or talk about this in front of strangers! What if someone recognised me from something and then the *Daily Mail* splashed me all over the front page? I guess this was the rainiest of days, then. (I would go on to find an OCD/ERP specialist later in the year. Again, privately. I would deplete all my savings entirely and, on top of having no maternity leave pay from an employer and Covid shutting down my industry, there wasn't much left in the coffers over the next year or so. Also, by being honest about my mental health struggles online, it definitely affected my job prospects.)

I had to talk about a trigger in therapy – so, nappy changing, for instance. I had to talk about why it bothered me so much. Then I had to try to *NOT* stop or neutralise the thought, which could be a physical compulsion, in the form of me shaking my head or clicking my fingers, or a mental one, like trying to think of something else or replace it with a 'happy thought'. This obviously didn't work as you can't do this eight times a minute for months on end. So, as my anxiety started to peak at the idea of doing something horrendous, and stopping the idea didn't work, I would ruminate. Internally I asked myself a thousand questions that could never have a definitive answer.

What if you do something inappropriate by accident?
I won't.
What if you do?
I don't think I will.
You don't THINK you will?
Well, I don't want to.
How do you know?
I don't KNOW, I just know.
What if you do it during a blackout and even you don't remember?
Well, I don't think that's likely!
But it's possible?
Yes, it's possible but . . .
So, you think you could possibly do something inappropriate?
Look, anything is possible but . . .

DEAR DIARY

Wow! Okay. So, you think it's possible – what does that say about you? There's a name for people like you!
I'm not that. I don't want to be that.
But you're not sure, are you?
I think I'm sure, I'm just so tired and I can't think straight.
Sounds like you need to take a step back just to protect the baby until you're sure.
Maybe you're right.
Get someone else to change him instead of you?
Yeah, okay, I could do with the breather.
So, you don't trust yourself?
No, I'm just a bit overwhelmed.
Overwhelmed with what? Being an abuser? Do you want to do it but can't admit it to yourself?
No, I feel disgusting just thinking about it.
How do you know?
What do you mean?
I mean, how do you know you're not enjoying it?
Because I'm not! I'm in tears, I'm shaking!
That could be excitement! You should check. Any feelings 'down there'?
What!?!?! No!
Have you checked!
I've checked in with 'down there' and I don't think so.
You don't think so? Check again!
I have but now I don't know if I actually felt something, or I just felt something because I engaged those muscles to check?
Sounds iffy to me!
I don't like this; I don't want this.

*Have you ever thought you could have split personalities? Maybe
you've been doing this the whole time and you just can't remember.*
I haven't!
Is this why you wanted a baby, so you could do this?
No, I love him. I just wanted a family.
You went to an awful lot of trouble with the IVF and everything.
That's because we wanted a baby!
Why?
I don't know.
You should check again to be sure.

And again. And again. And again. And again. And again. And again.

Eventually asking myself wasn't enough, it wasn't getting me anywhere, so I would usually turn to someone I trusted – namely my husband, but sometimes friends or family - and in a roundabout way, ask them instead. But not only did this push it from an unspoken theoretical into the real world, I had to wrestle with the idea that even discussing this would change how that person saw me forever. Maybe keep it to myself then.

Where were we?
You change him, I'll keep checking our groinal response or imagining him bloodied and battered on the floor after rolling off his changing mat.

Defeated, I would. A weakling, bullied and subdued by my own mind.

To say I was utterly beside myself with these exercises would be an understatement.

DEAR DIARY

My therapist suggested I start trying to order my thoughts to get some kind of a handle on them. Fuck me. Now I was supposed to leave a paper trail to be used against me when I was arrested or sectioned, or my husband was fighting for custody during our inevitable divorce?

Okay. I'd try anything at this point.

I bought an old school exercise book from WHSmith on my local high street (it's gone now). It was purple with three empty lines on the cover for me to write my name, class and subject, presumably. I hoped to find the purple calming. This did *not* work. I wrote 'Brain Journal' across the front and underlined it. Let's see if I could write my way out of this.

On the first page I dutifully wrote down what I'd been learning in therapy. Rules of engagement, so to speak.

1. They are <u>intrusive</u> thoughts

2. They are <u>automatic</u>

3. <u>Allow</u> the thoughts into your mind

4. Let them <u>stay</u> there

5. <u>Expect</u> them to come back

The following are all the entries I made, word for word. I was religious about it each night, getting into the bed that had once been my sanctuary and now felt like a pit of despair. I've redacted the names of specific medications; as I've mentioned, I have no medical training and type and dosage benefits can differ from patient to patient. I even used people's initials – feeling somehow I owe them that anonymity. A strange act of love to distance themselves from me. Though I know with every fibre of my being that each would be offended at the gesture and would proudly and wholly stand by my side. I just didn't know that then.

Here goes – and a little word of warning: it's a rocky ride.

<u>Wednesday 17 February 2021 (9:28pm)</u>
Mood: Low/anxious
Positives today:
- *Enjoyed watching* Death in Paradise *with T (my son)*
- *Felt less overwhelmed at his jabs this time round*
- *Really like taking him to D & E's (my in-laws) – feel more grounded in reality and I have to put a front on, which sometimes helps*

The horrible thoughts still stream in my mind all day long. I'm getting really fed up of them, which is a positive, I guess – I'd rather be angry at them than frightened. Keep trying to use E's (my counsellor) techniques when I get overwhelmed or suddenly anxious – FIND THE CORE OF THE ONION!

Seems to always come back to the same things. I'm afraid I'll end up alone. I'm afraid of being in trouble. I'm afraid I'm not good enough.

I wish I could believe these thoughts aren't real. But I can't. They feel so real. They're not just in my mind but in my body now too. I've thought/dreamt/worried about nothing else for months.

Gone up to 100mg and stopped taking ▮▮▮▮▮ *– let's hope it helps.*

I'm fighting every day but right now I'm feeling like a horrible wife and mother. This isn't fair on C (my husband) and being around T is simultaneously wonderful and excruciatingly uncomfortable.

Nightmare again last night. All the same themes. CSA and I (Child Sexual Assault and Incest – couldn't even write those words back then). *Makes me feel rotten and disgusting inside and out.*

Intention for tomorrow: *Let the thoughts wash over you and don't react.*

Friday 19 February 2021 (10:33pm)
Mood: Lighter/jittery
Positives today:
- T turned four months old
- Getting easier to be more tactile with T
- Thoughts were fewer today

A good day. Not great or normal, but I could still keep my brain in check. Still not great when I first wake up, especially after having horribly sexual or violent dreams – I'm quite disorientated. Getting up with T and going down for coffee and cleaning up helps to ground me.

Felt a little manic/jittery today – I know it's just my body adjusting to the new meds. I'm missing the relaxation element from the sedative. Guided sleep meditation NOT helping/working.

I have two self-tapes to work on over the weekend – which has focused me rather than panicked me. I'm still getting very overwhelmed by things. Need to go back to taking each day as it comes but worry I'm taking too long to get better.

T is so lovely. I love making him laugh. We even had a nap

together earlier and while I was quite tense and overly vigilant, it's not something I could have done a few weeks ago.

Got an email from my friend about PMS/breastfeeding nutrition. Made me feel anxious and inadequate that I'm not still b/feeding. I worry we're missing a connection but don't think I could have done it when I was really bad or taken the medication and I guess as long as he's fed and happy, it's more important that I get better.

Intention for tomorrow: Feel confident in something.

Saturday 20 February 2021 (6:27pm)

Mood: Manic/unfocused
Positives today:
- *Feeling more normal with everyone at D & E's*
- *Knowing I can talk to C*

Feeling very manic this afternoon. Like there are thirty different radio stations on in my head at once. I was okay at D & E's for the get-together but it was so noisy maybe I didn't notice the noise in my head. I feel extremely uncomfortable to be around T when other people are there. Like I'm under a microscope. Rationally, I know I'm not but everyone else just seems so much more casual and comfortable around my son than I am. Even writing 'my son' makes me feel anxious. It doesn't feel real and makes me feel guilty and gross that I would have such thoughts about a baby. He doesn't feel like <u>my</u> baby yet. I hope this will come with time. And all of this will be a distant memory. I keep picturing the summer in our garden and T splashing in a pool naked and laughing like kids are supposed to. My skin becomes so hot and tingly, and I feel so anxious and hyper aware. I hope this goes!!

DEAR DIARY

C suggests I take a ▓▓▓▓▓ as maybe this mania is just due to the higher dose of ▓▓▓▓▓. Hope so. I do feel a little quieter just under an hour after taking it.

Can't focus on anything. Can't physically relax my muscles. I'm so uptight.

This was how it all started to get bad a few weeks ago.

<u>SO</u> ready for this to be all over!!!!

PS (10:53pm) Read lots online about post partum OCD. It helps a bit but need to believe it's an illness, <u>not me</u>!

<u>Sunday 21 February 2021 (11:22pm)</u>
Mood: Lighter but still manic
Positives today:
- *Enjoy coffee and toast with T each morning watching* Death in Paradise
- *Spending time with A (brother), N (sister-in-law) and the kids (my niece and nephew)*
- *Easier being around T*

I'm pretty wired at the moment, seems to happen about 4-5 hours after taking 100mg ▓▓▓▓▓ It feels like every muscle in my body is tense and the signal to relax isn't getting there from my brain. Jammed frequencies. My sleep isn't great and I don't wake rested.

Weirdly, I'm SO mentally restless that I can't linger on any one thought. It's more like a bouncing echo.

Read today on OCD.UK about arousal anxiety and how it's normal and it's just because I'm monitoring and sensitising myself. I just think I'm so tense and anxious, everything is squeezed, and reality has become distorted. It made me feel better. I do feel like my forcefield is getting stronger with the help of my meds.

Did a self-tape today and things nearly felt normal. A bit of space from T helped gain perspective too.

I'm so tense right now, writing this, it feels as though my bones could shatter.

A better day and I can start to see how things will lift in the future. Much better than exactly a month ago when I had to be sedated.

Intention for tomorrow: Yoga practice.

Monday 22 February 2021 (10:09pm)
Mood: Lighter/anxious
Positives today:
- Sunshine
- Thoughts not so bad
- Agents liked my (audition) tapes

Best day so far, I think. Enjoyed being with T, persevered through the tough moments and the thoughts were spaced out. They're still pretty intense and visceral but each day gets a little easier.

The weather helped a lot. And getting out of the house.

I realised something today. It sounds so pseudo-shrinkish **BUT** I realised I need to give myself permission to be T's mother. It sounds so simple. I AM his mother, but I subconsciously haven't been allowing myself to be his parent in different senses of the word. Like I didn't have the authority, somehow. Constantly feel like I should be asking permission to do things or that cwtching and kissing him is inappropriate because he is someone else's child.

Maybe because of the thoughts I have been protecting him (and myself), but since he was born, I haven't given myself permission to become his mam. It's been a big part of struggling since his birth.

I did yoga today, which helps. The meds made me less manic today. Sleep is still crap, so C went out to get me something.

I would need fifty of these books to say how amazing C is/has been. Can't believe how lucky I am.

Intention for tomorrow: Own being T's mother*.

**Realise I don't like writing the word 'mother'. I hesitated every time. Must be a throwback to my childhood. (I'd had a very difficult and strained relationship with my mother).*

Tuesday 23 February 2021 (4:00pm)
Mood: Extremely edgy

Just waiting for my therapy session with E to start – feeling super jittery, tense and on edge.

These drugs are making me hyper and unfocused and (literally couldn't focus enough to finish that sentence).

Good session with E. Hard to focus at times and not sure I 'got' it until the end but the thought record was interesting and helpful. Explained why my responses to things are so disproportionate. The stakes are always so high for me.

Positives today (10:09pm)
- *Had a good nap with T (not fully relaxed) but liked being with him*
- *Pushed through my anxiety to do self-tape*
- *Felt more like T's mam*

I really can't wait for this whole nightmare to be over. I feel like I'm in some parallel timeline where nothing is quite right. Like there's been a huge shift. It's unsettling. So terrified of not getting better at all/quick enough.

C has been amazing. I can't believe his patience. From the outside, it must be so frustrating and annoying to see. Nothing has happened. Why can't I just snap out of it? But C has been nothing but supportive, kind and gentle. He knows me better than I know myself – if not for him keeping me grounded in some sense of reality, I couldn't have survived.

So worried there are lasting repercussions to this whole episode. C says not. Hope the ▆▆▆▆▆ *side effects wear off soon. I'm so tense, my bones might crack.*

Intention for tomorrow: Have fun!

<u>Weds 24 February 2021 (9:02pm)</u>
Mood: Blacker/v. tense
Positives today:
- *Things felt more like normal life around G & L (different niece and nephew)*
- *Did another self-tape*
- *T & C* ♥♥♥

Terrible sleep again. My body is so rigid and tensed up, it feels like I'll snap. I recognise this feeling from a few weeks ago when we first upped my ▆▆▆▆ *but the intrusive thoughts were so tense, I just linked it to that. It's like trying to sleep in a foxhole from* Band of Brothers *– I'm completely alert and hypervigilant.*

I've taken 4mg ▆▆▆▆ *– not feeling anything yet. My feet,* all day, have felt like they're curling upwards – like the witch in The Wizard of Oz.

Started to believe the thoughts are true again. It's so real. So graphic. All my feelings are in a tangle.

PNMH are useless – couldn't get in touch with Dr ▪▪, so they advised I go through my GP. Dr ▪▪▪▪ was great and we agreed I'm one week down, one week to go for the side effects.

God, I hope this helps and it's worth it. I'm absolutely exhausted. Every day is a living nightmare. I'm proud of myself for learning not to react at the thoughts but the darkness has such a strong pull on me.

If it's all true there is no hope for me, I'd rather take myself out of the equation than hurt C & T. I can't bear it. WHEN WILL THIS END?!?!?!!?

Intention for tomorrow: Stay busy and do some cleaning.

Thursday 25 February 2021 (8:54pm)
Mood: DARK
Positives today:
- Nice weather
- Everyone thinks I'm getting better

I'm struggling. It's all day, every day. When I'm talking to people. When I'm doing chores, when I'm watching TV. It's the enjoyment element. I don't know if it's real. I'm going through the motions so people don't worry about me, but I feel dead on the inside.

I really believe it could be true and I guess the only thing for me to decide is whether I can live with that.

I'm feeding my gorgeous, healthy baby boy and I'm thinking the most abhorrent things.

I can't take much more.

I'm exercising, taking my pills, I'm getting up and dressed. I spend all day with T, I'm writing in this journal, I'm having therapy, I'm speaking to PNMH, the GP, C and NOTHING IS WORKING!

What is wrong with me? Why am I so sick?

I just want to enjoy my family – but I guess I don't deserve to.

I've taken 4mg of ▮▮▮▮ *(1 hour ago) and I can't unclench my feet.*

I feel disgusting, inside and out.

I just want this to end.

Intention for tomorrow: Keep pretending.

Friday 26 February 2021 (4:14am)
Mood: Resigned

Can't sleep. Every muscle is tense. My mind won't stop. I'm losing faith. C & T are fast asleep – I wish I wasn't ruining their lives. I'd rather be a dead mother than a bad mother.

I can't go on like this.

Every day. For months. Every minute of every day.

I keep wishing I could go back to being pregnant before I ruined everything.

I should tell C but there's only so much he can put up with.

All of the healthcare people are beyond useless – I've reached the limit of their care.

There is no hope for me.

Got up with T. Had our usual morning: breakfast and Death in Paradise. *Asked C to take him out to Dad's. Couldn't face it and needed time to myself.*

DEAR DIARY

Took 2mg of ▇▇▇ at 11:30 and had a really good sleep. Just a shame I woke up.

My reactions are slowly killing me. It makes me sick not knowing if I like the feelings. I don't know.

Endless streams of horrid thoughts and images. Don't bother leaving the house. I'm sick of trying and I feel better for it.

T is happy and healthy and that's the best I can do.

A deep sleep that doesn't end is the nicest thought I've had all day.

Intention for tomorrow: ?

Saturday 27 February 2021 (10:22pm)

Mood: Lighter/hopeful

Positives today:
- The weather is really helping
- T rolled over!!!
- Sunset walk with Bob

Something is shifting. Everything is still happening but it's panicking me less. It's horrible to have lovely moments with T and be bombarded with disgusting images and feelings.

Since I've given in and I'm not fighting them, it's become easier.

Sleep is the answer too! Good nap yesterday then a full night's sleep (with ▇▇▇) has made a huge difference.

I think when this is behind me, I will come to realise how incredibly ill I was becoming. Maybe my past mental health stuff and the episode in Stratford were a blessing in disguise. I knew something was wrong a lot sooner.

From all my reading and research, I was clearly on my way

to postpartum psychosis. I should have told C more about my symptoms. I was hallucinating (I just thought I was tired). I believed this terrible thing was true and even had concocted fake memories of it.

I have been terrified of T since the moment he was born. Being near him felt like I was drowning. That first night in hospital, when he was in SCBU and I went to my bed on the ward, once I lay down I was paralysed with fear. I didn't move. I lay on my back for about six hours straight, silently crying, wishing I could go back to being pregnant like I was the day before. It got worse from there.

It's hard to write but I must get it all out of my brain and one day tell C the whole truth.

I planned to die. I found a place and chose a date (31st Jan) – it gave me five days to get everything ready so C & T were taken care of. I tried to get life insurance but they don't pay out for suicide in the first 12 months. It would be the last day of the month (neater). It would (and did) snow. I would call the emergency services just before. I thought this was the best plan. I had found a secluded spot so no dangers of strangers finding me and I would **NEVER** do that to C. Paramedics are used to seeing dead bodies and I would have ID and a note in my pocket, so he wouldn't have to identify me.

It brought such a sense of calm over me for days. I'd had no peace and suddenly there was an end in sight. I wasn't scared at all. It was the best thing I could do. The drugs started working a few days later and lifted me enough to put my plan on hold and I selfishly wanted more time with C & T. My mind was entirely broken and stuck on repeat.

I thought I was a danger to my baby – what else could I do?

DEAR DIARY

Nothing has been like I thought it would be. I thought I would be a natural mother and that the bond would be instant. I thought I would be afraid of dying. I thought I couldn't love C more but then he saved me again.

Streams of images and constant monitoring for reactions continue. I hope they end soon.

I hope I'm truly not a monster. I don't want to be a monster.

Intention for tomorrow: <u>One day at a time.</u>

Sunday 28 February 2021

Mood: Calmer

Positives today:
- Spending lots of time with T
- Sunshine
- Gorgeous walk with C & T
- Fewer thoughts

I've turned a corner! I don't want to jinx it but today has been the quietest my brain has been for months. The thoughts were there but didn't land or have as much impact or meaning.

I watched a video last night where two women discussed OCD and intrusive thoughts and it helped me **so** much.

I also think the drugs are starting to help.

Together, it's giving me perspective.

I'm absolutely terrified of being 'struck down' again by my brain. Both C & E [therapist] think I need to not think of it as some mystical, malevolent force over which I have no control. It's a nice idea but hard in practice.

My memory of this time is so blurry. I think this is because 1) it's a symptom of PND [postnatal depression] and 2) it was *so traumatic, my brain blocked it out. Not remembering how it started scares me as it means I can't prevent it from happening in the future.*

In the meantime, I will enjoy being with my little boy while the 'brain peace' lasts. It was so weird how today, all of that uncomfortable and tormented feeling was largely gone and I felt like me again. I felt like a natural with my baby. Fingers crossed it continues although I can't do any superstitious things anymore as they fuel my OCD. (Sidenote: I had always knocked on wood if I said something bad, which morphed into me knocking on my forehead when I thought something bad, or saluting magpies, or not walking on cracks in the pavement – habits I had always performed were now scrupulously adhered to, as the consequences could be dire for my baby.)

Intention for tomorrow: Start running again.

Monday 1 March (10:16pm)
Mood: Better but still down
Positives today:
- *Loved being around T*
- *Start of spring*
- *Reading at bedtime with T*

It felt like a step backwards today but trying not to let it derail me. I think it's just because I woke in the middle of the night and I know it sounds stupid but C had come to bed later and somehow we swapped back to our original sides, so I was next to T again (we had swapped sides of the bed so my husband could tend to the baby in the night and give me a break).

DEAR DIARY

And it just panicked me. I was back in those weeks where I was so scared of the baby, I was paralysed in the dark.

The more I read, the more convinced I am that I had the beginnings of psychosis. I was absolutely **CONVINCED** *that I was an evil, murderous child molester and I had to die to be stopped. I keep reading about women who truly believed alternate realities that were so far removed from their life or who they were. Another symptom is being terrified of your baby. I absolutely was. It's hard to explain but being around him felt like I couldn't breathe. Also, my hearing became muted and I had tunnel vision. This is what I meant when I said I felt like I was behind thick glass or underwater. These aren't symptoms of simple postnatal OCD or PND. My entire reality shifted and it's v. v. slowly shifting back to normal.*

I don't need to be apart from T. I need to be near him, no matter how uncomfortable it is/was.

Dad hasn't asked me how I am. Nor has S (sister-in-law). This disappoints me but doesn't make me upset. (Turns out they didn't want to ask me how I was so as not to upset me but were checking in with my husband every day.)

I'm so tired from all this. I'm sick of being me. I'd love to be knocked out and sleep for two whole days.

Intention for tomorrow: Write a paragraph for IVF sitcom.

Tuesday 2 March 2021 (10:34pm)
Mood: More normal
Positives today:
- Sunny, peaceful walk with Bob and T
- Seeing N (my sister-in-law) and her loving the new coat I got her
- Meds are working

Today was interesting. I think a lot of my worry and depression stems from the feeling of how awful it was a few weeks ago and the fear of feeling it again.

The sunshine helps so much.

I had a little walk earlier on top of the mountain. At first it was a nightmare: T was screaming in his carrier, I was too hot in a thick, woolly jumper, Bob was pulling too hard and my shoelace got caught and I nearly fell over with the baby!! But then I took a deep breath and carried on. It was so peaceful and sunny. I saw some rabbits! T stopped crying, Bob listened to me, and I felt more grounded.

I had a good session with E.

The 'evidence' part of the thought sheet was a huge revelation. She bluntly asked me 'how many children have you hurt to date?' I know it's stupid – because it's rationally obvious – but I felt such overwhelming relief when I said 'none' out loud.

'How many children are you planning to hurt in the future?'

'None.'

I cried. There was no 'evidence' for any of these thoughts and it's the first time I <u>got</u> that! There's still doubt and fear but I'm going to work so hard to shift how I feel about how I think and vice versa.

Intention for tomorrow: Drift through the day.

Wednesday 3 March 2021 (9:42pm)

Mood: Listless
Positives today:
- *Lovely time with T*
- *Washed my hair*

Today was interesting. It's been dark and rainy, and I didn't leave the house. I think I wanted a day of not pretending. My mind is so unfocused. Can't learn lines, couldn't face a self-tape.

Me and C have been very distant over the past few days. I think I withdrew from him as the side effects made me worse and then he withdrew because of that. I think he's had enough. These past 7–8 weeks have been tough on him and I know he aches all day (fibromyalgia). I think I'm too scared to ask what's wrong in case he says it's me. He has witnessed an intensely dark side to me and maybe it's changed how he sees me. Maybe he's just tired. Neither of us were prepared for T turning our lives completely upside down. It's just been the two of us for sixteen years and then we were given this scary Tamagotchi.

I know we'll find our stride.

I'm trying so hard to get better.

T is beautiful and adorable and C understands me better than I understand myself – so why is it still so hard?

There's a disconnection – still – BUT the thoughts were much easier and less impactful today and I love being tactile with T now.

Work is stressing me too. If I can't cope while we're all in lockdown and there's nowhere I have to be, what will it be like if I get a job and have to go back to real life like this?

Intention for tomorrow: <u>FOCUS</u>

Thursday 4 March 2021 (10:12pm)

Mood: Scared/stuck

Positives today:
- Enjoyed taking T to D & E's
- Changed the bed and dusted
- C was happy doing some gardening

I wish this alternate reality would end. I hope this is temporary, otherwise this nightmarish state of mind is my new normal. I took T to 'the spot' today. It was hard but I needed to do it to realise how far I've come in five weeks. I felt better.

I'm in such a fugue. But it's all so contradictory. I feel dog-tired but I'm hyperalert. I enjoy being with T but I find it intensely uncomfortable at times. I feel extremely close and really distant from C, all at the same time.

I think deep down, I'm scared. Terrified, actually. And just plain sad. I know it's part hormonal/part chemical/part PTSD from how dangerously ill I was a few weeks ago. It's like I'm walking around with a ticking time bomb inside my head. I don't know when/if my mind is going to attack me again.

I also feel deeply ashamed and until I can forgive myself or understand that none of this was ever real, I'll never move on. I feel like I've failed T and he's only been here for nineteen weeks. How will I ever make it up to him?

Will I ever feel like myself again?

When will I feel safe again?

Work and sex have started to stress me, too. I feel so inadequate. So rubbish, in terms of my career and worried I can never be like 'that' again with C again after everything I've thought and told him. Aaaaaaaaagggggggghhhhhhhhhhhhhh.

Intention for tomorrow: Don't second-guess.

<u>Friday 5 March 2021 (3:52am)</u>
Can't sleep.
Can't believe it's not true.
It's destroying me.
*I **hate** this!!!!*

DEAR DIARY

(12:04 am)
Mood: Steadier
Positives today:
- *Seeing L (nephew)*
- *Calmer thoughts*

Today was better than expected! Again, the sunshine helps. I didn't sleep v. well but realised getting up and facing my fear was better than worryingly trying to sleep. I did have a little nap this afternoon with T. It was lovely. I'm feeling a little less overwhelmed and frightened each day. It's not so much him but the situation that scares me. The overwhelming responsibility has knocked me sideways from day one and I never expected it to. He's such a lovely little boy and he's changing all the time.

*I think I need to forgive myself for everything that's happened. Or rather **not** happened.*

It's a relatively short amount of time and as quickly as I went down, I'm coming back up. I keep clinging to something C said weeks ago: not only does he know I'll get better, but I'll be better than before. I have learnt a lot in the last few months. About my fears, my brain chemistry, my capacity to trust C, when I couldn't trust myself or basic reality and I'm proud of myself for continuing to love and care for T when the fabric of my mind was torn apart.

I need to move on now.
Enough.
Intention for tomorrow: Time with my boys.

SHE SEEMS FINE TO ME

<u>Sunday 7 March 2021(11:36am)</u>
Didn't write anything last night for the first time in weeks. I forgot – which is maybe a good sign? I was also exhausted and sleep isn't that restful at the moment.

I'm very confused about how I feel and which feelings to trust. Which thoughts are intrusive and which are just me?

I'm holding myself back from T because I'm absolutely petrified of what will happen if I fully bond with him and let myself feel the full extent of my emotion for him. A lot of this is subconscious and automatic. A self-protection mechanism. But it hurts my heart to look at him sometimes and not feel it all.

Taking Bob for a walk. Need some time to myself.

(10:43pm)
Mood: Despondent
Positives today:
- *Good walk with Bob*
- *T laughing*
- *Nice nap with T*

I'm <u>still</u> struggling. I want to feel comfortable in my own body again. This is so hard and so frustrating because NOTHING has/is happening. It's all of my own making. But I feel wretched in the truest sense of the word.

Months of non-stop, obsessive, obscene thinking. I'm missing out on precious time with T. He's growing so fast and I'm ruining it.

Health visitor is coming tomorrow – pointless. Will fake being better so we can knock those visits on the head. At this point they're just counterproductive. She makes me feel worse.

DEAR DIARY

I feel like the meds have helped but mainly with my outward symptoms. I feel like I'm in a glass box screaming and no one can hear me anymore.

Intention for tomorrow: RUN!

Monday 8 March 2021 (11:13pm)
Mood: OK
Positives today:
- T being a tiny genius in the bath
- Walk in the sunshine with C, T & Bob
- Harry and Meghan interview

We just finished watching the H & M interview with Oprah on TV. C thinks it's mainly bollocks, but I believe them, even if they can be a bit cringe. But one thing really resonated with me. When Meghan was talking about feeling suicidal, I completely and utterly believed her because the state of mind she described and the methodical nature of the thinking is exactly *how I felt*. Feeling TRULY suicidal is not what you imagine it to be. It's not dramatic or emotional or even poignant — it's very simple and quiet. It makes perfect sense at the time. There are a thousand insurmountable problems and suddenly a very easy answer solves all of them. It feels like a kindness. Almost a duty or service. It's hard to explain unless you've wholly decided to do it and that's why I believed her. It also really helped that she talked about it and made me feel less mental and defective.

I enjoy being with T **so** much, even with the constant barrage of intrusive thoughts and feelings. I can't imagine how wonderful it will feel when it's simply the nice stuff.

I'm very afraid that I'm just going to have to learn to live with this, like I do now, and the challenge will be not believing the thoughts and letting them stream without paying too much attention. It's miserable but doable, I think.

I'd love it to stop though.

Intention for tomorrow: V/O sample for J (voiceover agent).

PS Had a PNMH call and H/V visit – both fucking useless and left me feeling like shit.

Tuesday 9 March 2021 (11:06pm)
Mood: Getting there
Positives today:
- Walk with C, T, Bob and D & E
- Great session with E on Zoom
- Easier with T

Wasn't sure how today would pan out. Not getting v. restful sleep BUT getting out of the house was a good idea. I'm always better when I'm around D & E – they keep me grounded without really trying. They remind me who I used to be.

We had a lovely walk together along the Taff Trail. T sat facing out of his carrier while C carried him and T's face is so lovely to watch as he takes everything in.

Sometimes when I have ten mins where I don't think of him or I haven't looked at him, I feel like such a terrible mother, but I think that comes under the 'unrealistic expectations of motherhood' thing that E talked about. I'm glad we spent the session talking about how and why things are better and also what's holding me back.

1) I'm terrified of going back into that dark, hopeless nightmare of a time.
2) While I'm getting my head around 'they're just thoughts', I'll never move on until I understand 'they're just feelings' as well. I thought any sensation or sensitising was evidence that the thoughts were real but E says its common and only evidence that I have a NORMAL HUMAN BODY! FEELINGS ARE NOT FACTS.

It's really helped and I've felt lighter all evening. C is so understanding and non-judgemental – I don't know how or why he does it. But not having to hide a single thing from him is the single most important thing for my recovery. I'm proud of myself for bringing it up with E and she's reassured me (for now!). Need to write a list of what's different now to when I was at my worst and why it won't happen that intensely again.

Intention for tomorrow: Be in the present.

Wednesday 10 March 2021 (10:38pm)
Mood: Getting there (a bit more)
Positives today:
- T laughing
- Crossword with C
- Happy Mum, Happy Baby podcast

Today was good. I think I've turned another corner. Therapy really helped yesterday, and I've been on 100mg ▮▮▮▮▮▮ for three weeks today. I'm evening out! I can go for longer periods without the thoughts and a lot of the time, it's me remembering to have them.

T is changing so much every day. He's so lovely. My thoughts and feelings are still too clouded. I think I'm having a lot of very nice, natural thoughts and feelings but I've spent so long 'sinisterising' them – it'll take me a while to shift my thinking.

I think that's a big thing for me. Time. It will just take time.

I worry I've done irreparable damage but I have to hope that's not true. I also have to be brave and stop seeking reassurance, as it's a compulsion and only a temporary fix. Don't feed the doubt monster!!! I've also stopped other tics as much as possible i.e. touching wood for luck, clicking, shaking my head to get rid of thoughts, etc. I'm still body-checking but from today, I'm trying to observe it and let it pass.

Listening to the Happy Mum, Happy Baby podcast was actually really helpful. It was with Kate Middleton and they talked a lot about unrealistic expectations of motherhood and even having thoughts you may think means they'll take your baby away.

I can't imagine how wonderful it would be to just enjoy T. For me to just be in the moment and enjoy him laughing or making funny noises (like I always have with my nieces and nephews). I do enjoy it but it's in tandem with a nightmare.

Intention for tomorrow: Text K [producer] about IVF sitcom.

<u>Thursday 11 March 2021 (12:06am)</u>
Mood: A step backwards
Positives today:
- *Seeing L [nephew]*
- *Reading more articles about intrusive thoughts*
- *Thinking of a future holiday*

Today started off tough. The nasty side effect of my feet and lower legs cramping started up in the night. It makes my body so incredibly clenched and tense — feels like my bones will break. Hope it goes soon.

Had two hours' sleep this morning, so C took T but I need to avoid becoming overtired. I'm glad I slept a little but even with 2mg ▮▮▮▮ I was so tense and had bad dreams. It puts me on a darker path.

Really proud of myself for getting up and out and changing my state of mind.

Worried D & E are getting annoyed with me turning up every day but I find it so helpful.

I'm not getting enough exercise. Need to start running again and do yoga — I don't feel like it but it helps.

Still not quite believing this is all a condition and that I'm not actually a complete freak.

JUST NEED TIME!!!!!

Want to enjoy my gorgeous baby without any malevolent feelings!

Intention for tomorrow: NEW DAY.

Saturday 13 March 2021 (10:34pm)

Mood: Disappointed and defeated
Positives today:
- *Extra sleep*
- *Crossword with C*
- *Walk with T and Bob*

Every day feels like one step forward and two steps back. Just when I think I've got a handle on it and I'm moving on, it comes thundering back. Tonight, it's been very intense and vivid again. I think watching Line of Duty didn't help — it's quite anxiety-inducing and darkly sexual sometimes, which makes me very confused.

What is the difference between intrusive thoughts and wants or desires? The thing that scares me the most is am I actually all these terrible things but because I know it's wrong, I'd never do anything?? Or is my mind broken and playing tricks on me??

I guess that's why OCD is called the Doubting Disease in France.

I feel like the life I'm living isn't right. I know that lockdown and having a baby are making things feel surreal, but I can't seem to get a foothold in reality. My whole day is spent fighting to keep my mind straight and caring for T. That's why the house is a tip and I can barely fit a walk in with Bob.

I HATE these 'feelings'!!! Are they real? I guess I won't get better until I stop asking that question.

This time last year, I remember thinking that next Mother's Day, I would be a mother and everything would be complete. I don't feel complete — I feel broken and I'm dreading tomorrow as I don't deserve to celebrate Mother's Day. Nothing is as it should be.

Intention for tomorrow: Remember what you've learnt.

PS No booze tomorrow.

DEAR DIARY

<u>Sunday 14 March 2021 (9:38pm)</u>
Mood: Sad and scared
Positives today:
- *Mother's Day?*
- *Being around everyone again*
- *Sorting out T's clothes*

I found today hard. I felt like a fraud.

C got me lovely presents and I had so many texts from people wishing me a happy first Mother's Day – but I just feel disgusting inside and out.

I feel rotten and dead inside. I want to enjoy T and to a certain extent, I do. But it's not full. It's not right. Every single day for months, my mind has been in this incredibly dark place but more than that, my body has not released or relaxed or felt normal since T was born.

I imagine him reading this when he's older and it fills me with shame.

I didn't deserve a Mother's Day today. I'm not getting better – I'm just much better at masking it and not reacting outwardly to what's happening in my mind.

No one at D & E's today would have had any idea that I just wanted to curl up and die.

When will this lift?

It's testament to how incredible T is that I want to be around him and he can make me laugh because it doesn't feel right or natural and I'm losing faith that there is <u>nothing</u> wrong with me.

I didn't sleep again last night. My body feels like pure rigor mortis and while C & T slept, I quietly cried because I'm living this nightmarish parallel life.

Intention for tomorrow: I just don't know.

Monday 15th March 2021 (10:03pm)
Mood: Very dark
Positives today:
- Sleep!
- Went for a run
- Walk with Bob & T

Why aren't my pills working??

Why aren't my strategies working??

Therapy, journalling, walks, talking about it, non-avoidance . . .

NOTHING IS WORKING!!!!!!

The only upside to the drugs is that I can't emotionally react to anything as much. I can look totally relaxed and normal and there's a fucking nightmare scrolling through my head and I can feel it surging through my body!

I can't keep living like this.

T is perfect and I'm completely miserable.

I can't talk to C – I feel too disconnected.

I'm fantasising about suicide again. I know, logically, that's a bad sign but it's the only thing that calms me. It's like an escape plan in my back pocket for when it's so exhaustingly relentless.

Took a sleeping pill and it obviously worked, had good, deep sleep – nearly made me forget.

I don't feel right!!!!!!!!!!!!!!

And there's nothing that can be done. I'm already doing everything available to me. PNMH ARE FUCKING USELESS.

DEAR DIARY

The new health visitor is nice but can't help me in any tangible way. Why do they think baby massage is the answer to any problem? Bewildering. The GP will just chop and change my meds and I can't face that.

My mind is diseased, and it feels inoperable. I'm even sabotaging myself. Work things I should have done/have promised to do – I'm purposely not doing them. I just don't care.

Look into TMS★ – expensive but worth a go??

Intention for tomorrow: <u>Don't wake up.</u>

★TMS, or Transcranial Magnetic Stimulation, is a non-invasive procedure that uses magnetic fields to stimulate specific areas of the brain.

<u>Tuesday 16 March 2021(1:53am)</u>
Mood: BLACK
Positives today:
- T
- Therapy

Today was a low point. It's been creeping up on me and it finally overwhelmed me.

C caught me crying. It feels so hopeless.

I really want it all to end.

I know T is here and he's safe and healthy and that C will do an amazing job with him – I have zero worries about them. I'm the danger. The bad influence in their lives.

Therapy helped a little but we were going around in circles. Black and white thinking, unrealistic expectations, low self-esteem are supposedly root causes but I'm worried that's all a lie and I'm as sinister and dark as I feel.

Glad I told E about the BBC article, though – maybe I should hand myself in to the police?! (Looking into this, I remembered it was an article I'd read that morning on the BBC News app – 'Online abuse – I found out that my husband had indecent images'.[4] *I was beside myself after another sleepless night and convinced myself that this article was really a portent about me, and that I should head to my local police station. 'And say what?' my husband would ask, kindly but with a heavy note of incredulity. 'I don't know – that this could be me too? I might be like this man, even though I don't want to be.')*

According to Dr ▮▮▮▮▮*, I just need to persevere with the 100mg and the* ▮▮▮▮ *will kick in soon!*

Who the hell knows?!?

I just need to make sure my boys are taken care of and that everything will be alright for them.

My mind is attacking me and I'm supposed to challenge it and look for evidence but I'm just so fucking tired.

Intention for tomorrow: Just enjoy time with C & T.

PS Period started today.

<u>Wednesday 17 March 2021 (10:55pm)</u>
Mood: END OF MY TETHER
Positives today:
- *Lovely walk with C & T in Llanwonno*
- *Seeing G & L helps me feel normal*
- *T laughing at peek-a-boo*

DEAR DIARY

I can't write the same things over and over. The thoughts and images are the same. Some days I can handle it, some days I can't, but it's always there.

I'm just going to write my base feelings:
- *Overwhelmed*
- *Hopeless*
- *Ashamed*
- *Frightened*
- *Disgusting*
- *Exhausted*
- *Out-of-step*
- *A failure*
- *Manic*
- *Tense*
- *Sad*

Reasons why my feelings are attached to my habitual thinking:
- *Black and white thinking*
- *All or nothing thinking*
- *Unrealistic expectations*
- *Self-esteem*

Fears arising from thoughts + feelings =
- *I'm a monster*
- *I'll be in trouble*
- *I'll be alone*
- *I'll do something irreparable*
- *I won't be able to live with myself*
- *I will die*

~~This is hard~~ I'm finding this hard because:
- I won't give myself a break
- I put too much pressure on myself
- I don't think I'm good enough
- I'm inherently evil

<u>Thursday 18 March 2021(1:13am)</u>
Mood: Frightened
Positives today:
- Good sleep this morning with T
- Nice walk

My grip on reality is really fragile. I can't remember what it's like to not be like this. To have a sense of peace — of joy.

My heart sinks fifty times a day.

It's so demoralising. I hate it. I want to feel normal again. I want to feel as if the world isn't ending, and the darkness won't completely envelop me. I want a sense of perspective. I want to know myself again. Not live in this perpetual, doubting, sinister nightmare. I've been trying to lean into it, not seek reassurance and use face-my-fear tactics but I'm still like this.

I need to try something new. I have another session with E tomorrow. Will try to get something more tangible to try.

I'm stuck. There's no way out. I can't leave as it would hurt C but staying is hurting me.

So worried I'm ruining T.

When will this nightmare end?

When will I feel peace again?!

Intention for tomorrow: <u>Tasks</u>. Keep busy.

Friday 19 March 2021 (1:00am)

Mood: Drained but hopeful

Today's positives:

- *Being honest with C*
- *Therapy*
- *Line of Duty finale*

<u>C is amazing!</u>

I can't understand for the life of me how he can be so understanding, non-judgemental, kind, patient and normal with me about a condition that is such a waste of time and not based in the real world.

But he knows it's real to me.

If I can get through this, I will understand myself so much better.

I have to keep coming back to <u>IT'S HOW I SEE MYSELF.</u>

Particular content of unwanted, obsessive thinking is irrelevant. It's confirmation bias for me that I'm a terrible person. A monster.

Until that shifts, my symptoms won't shift.

I feel incredibly guilty that I've ruined what should have been a magical time for us all. For C. But maybe it's never a 'magical' time for anyone – and that's part of my unrealistic expectations and black and white thinking.

I have to put this guilt aside and concentrate on just getting better. C wouldn't want me to waste energy on feeling bad for him – just focus on moving forward.

Hormones + chemicals + history + sleep deprivation + new responsibility + trauma = CURRENT OCD EPISODE

Intention for tomorrow: Forget symptoms, focus on core issues ⇒ SELF WORTH.

SHE SEEMS FINE TO ME

<u>Saturday 20 March 2021 (12:33am)</u>
Mood: Tired but brighter
Today's positives:
- *Seeing family*
- *Nap with T*
- *Normal Saturday night with C*

Today was mixed but I've come out of it feeling more positive.

I had more sleep, which always gives me more perspective.

I think I have to unashamedly sleep as much as possible – it really helps!

Whenever I wake, I get a huge surge of cortisol. It's so horrible.

I had a lovely nap with T – I didn't sleep very comfortably but he did and it was nice just to 'be' with him.

I need to get back on top of my fitness – it does help, even when I don't feel like it. I had shin splints for a few weeks and then a horribly heavy period – so starting Monday, back to running and yoga.

Feeling a surge of good energy, don't want to question it too much – maybe my meds are FINALLY helping (even though the side effects are still painful).

Intention for tomorrow: <u>Stay light</u>.

<u>Sunday 21 March 2021 (11:09am)</u>
Mood: ?
Positives today:
- *Good sleep*
- *Nice evening last night.*
- *Walk with C and H (nephew)*

DEAR DIARY

Today was good. Thoughts still pop up but I'm definitely body-checking less and dismissing it when I do. I've been feeling very embarrassed today. When I think of telling people what I've been thinking/worrying about, it's making me feel really ashamed.

I find it <u>way</u> easier to be with T now. He's just so lovely. I notice I feel it difficult to be around him when we're with other people – or more that I feel self-conscious of people judging how I am with him and tend to go the other way and be quite hands off. Maybe that's the same for all new parents, especially mothers as we're supposed to be naturals.

I'm getting really sick of feeling scared. Scared of the thoughts, scared they mean something, scared it'll get worse, scared it'll come back in the future and scared it'll never go away.

I want to live life again. Enjoy it and not just 'get through another day'.

Sleeping definitely helps – the more I get, the more even I am.

Real-world responsibilities are beginning to creep back in. I keep feeling like I'm letting people down or I'm not on the ball enough BUT I've been doing all my self-tapes (except those two or three when I was very unwell). Give yourself a break.

Intention for tomorrow: <u>ORGANISE!</u>

Monday 22 March 2021

Mood: Bright but edgy
Positives today:
- *Got lots of errands done*
- *Spoke to O (my agent)*
- *Sunshine*
- *Exercise*

It's now two months since the worst day, when I broke and had to be sedated. I'm a lot stronger and I know myself and my condition a lot more.

I'm still terrified it will come back but I have to stop thinking of 'it' as some sort of malevolent force that's out of my control. There were many contributing factors and I know the signs now.

I had a good sleep and the weather was lovely to wake up to. T is gorgeous now but just thinking/writing this made me feel sinister – I have to stop warping lovely thoughts and moments.

Did lots of organisational things today – which helped me feel more in control.

I think the meds are starting to work too (fingers crossed!!)

I really don't want to go down again – I can't take it.

I faced my fears and spoke to O today. I think I get so anxious because deep down I think I'm more trouble than I'm worth. It all comes back to <u>self-worth</u>. Change that thinking and everything else will shift.

Running and yoga helps too.

Best evening for thoughts and mood I've had for long time. It scares me how ill I was.

Worried about C's mood/health – all of this must have taken a toll. Calling the docs for him tomorrow.

Intention for tomorrow: Carefree.

<u>Tuesday 23 March 2021 (11:30pm)</u>
Mood: Bad sleep but better
Positives today:
- *Good therapy session*
- *Nice walk with C, Dad and T*

DEAR DIARY

Had a really bad night's sleep last night. My body is so tight and tense, I physically couldn't relax enough to sleep, even with a sleeping pill.

Got to sleep about 4:30am and then had restless sleep with lots of jolting awake. Went back to sleep at 10:30am – woke up at 12:30pm to find C and T gone. Really disorientating.

Dad was at D & E's too when I arrived at 1:30 to meet C & T and I just feel like they all think I'm a crap mum. I worry when T isn't my first thought when he's not with me. Maybe I just haven't known him long enough.

What was weirdly good about last night was that as buzzed and hyperalert as I was, the horrible, intrusive thoughts weren't really there. It was as if the disguise had gone and the actual root problem was revealed – which is intense anxiety and self-doubt. I want to feel better. I did for a short time earlier but then, weirdly, hearing from Zawe made me feel bad about myself. It's ten years since Fresh Meat *and I feel, out of all of us, my career has stalled and I'm scrabbling around for tiny parts. J & J are so successful, G works consistently, C is the lead in different shows and Z is always working and is now doing the next Marvel film. I'm so happy for them, I just wish it didn't highlight my failures to me so much. BUT I have an amazing husband, a lovely home, Bob, and T is the baby we always wanted* ♥

Intention for tomorrow: <u>Focus on work</u>.

<u>Wednesday 24 March 2021 (10:36pm)</u>
Mood: More focused
Positives today:
- *Sunshine*
- *Busy all day*
- *Time with T*

Today was a good day! I still had moments of excessive worry and self-doubt, and I was knackered after a couple of crappy sleeps BUT we all got up early. C had work and I had lots to accomplish today – it was good to get organised and stay busy.

I did work for self-tapes, went for a run, took T and Bob for a walk in the sunshine. C was working – which I know is making him feel better.

It's the easiest I've felt around T – he's such a joy ♥

He had his third set of jabs today and when I think of how I've improved with each visit, I'm proud of myself.

I've even been doing stuff for the NAS (National Autistic Society – I'm an ambassador) too. One day at a time. Enjoying each little moment with T.

Due to lockdown, the one upside is that there's nothing to do except simple things. Walks, watching TV with C, time with T, D & E.

Looks like I've got restless leg syndrome (RLS) – which helps me feel less mad and like I'm having unprecedented side effects.

The meds are certainly helping with mood, I think. Plus, exercise and therapy.

Today <u>almost</u> felt like real life. Almost. It's more the shadow or echo of the bad thoughts and how poorly I really was.

DEAR DIARY

T has been a little unwell tonight — due to his jabs — which isn't like him. But it cemented in my mind that there isn't anything I wouldn't do to stop him from hurting.

Intention for tomorrow: Self-tapes and T.

Thursday 25 March 2021 (11:14pm)

Mood: Productive

Positives today:
- Got back in touch with the NAS
- Did 3 x self-tapes
- Signed up to do a 7k run for NAS
- T and sunshine

Today was a good day. Getting much more perspective. I'm still highly anxious and physically vigilant but the iron tablets seem to be working for the RLS. Slept a bit better and even though I had a lot on and felt overwhelmed, I used the techniques E had discussed with me.

Trying to work on underlying feelings of inadequacy and general 'bad-person-ness'.

T has been really grizzly — I think it's the jabs. D seemed in a bad mood earlier — I'm trying to make sure I don't read too much into it, that maybe he's sick of having me around all the time. I'm sure it's nothing to do with me but I'll give them a day off tomorrow. Really need to clean the house — it should help declutter my mind.

I'd been doing really well all day but then had a funny hour just now. I think any time anything comes up about sex or I think about anything like that while I'm with T, I feel sinister and inappropriate. Need to separate the two.

Really sick of this warped thinking. Want to enjoy lovely T with no strings attached.

Signed up to run 7k for the NAS. Think it will be a really good challenge for me. I'd love to accomplish it. At least then I'll feel like I've done one good thing.

⇒ *Bad thinking – challenge it.*
Evidence you've done anything 'bad' = **NONE**
Intention for tomorrow: Organise.

THINGS TO REMEMBER IN DARK MOMENTS
  1) Talk about it.
  2) Challenge your thoughts
  3) You are safe.
  4) It won't last forever.
  5) Go for a walk/run/coffee.

Every 3–4 weeks your hormones make you feel at ROCK BOTTOM! You're not!

<u>Monday 29th March 2021 (11:01pm)</u>
Mood: Confused again
Positives today:
  - *Ran 4k*
  - *Walked Bob and T*
  - *Did yoga*

I haven't written over the weekend mainly because I was exhausted when I got into bed and also because I'm losing faith that writing all this helps.

DEAR DIARY

I had a little setback on Saturday night. T wouldn't stop crying and I just felt so exhausted from no/strained sleep that I burst into tears. C made me take a ▮▮▮▮▮▮ (15mg). I was out for fourteen hours but felt sluggish today.

I've had another weird setback this evening with the sudden 'knowledge' that the dreams/thoughts must be true again. I find it hard to think or feel anything remotely sexual when the baby is anywhere near me. I find it highly inappropriate. But I guess I'm only human and haven't had sex for 9–10 months, which after years of regular sex for 'trying' is another adjustment. I just dread having sex again and having intrusive thoughts and it freaking me out so much I go back to square one.

Feeling horrible right now, finding it difficult to have perspective and not believe the bad thoughts to be real when they manifest as 'feelings'.

I've read stories from people in my situation to remind me – I'm not shying away from T (he's in bed next to me) and I've just read my golden rules.

IT IS NOT REAL.

THEY ARE INTRUSIVE THOUGHTS.

Intention for tomorrow: Keep challenging thoughts!

Weds 31 March 2021 (11:22pm)

Mood: Conflicted

Positives today:
- *Ran over 5k*
- *Sunshine*
- *Pizza with C*
- *Playing with T*

I didn't write again last night. Maybe that's a good sign?

I've been increasing my running distance each day, so I'm exhausted by bedtime. I did nearly 20,000 steps yesterday.

Just had a bit of a meltdown with C. It's the first time I really 'saw' that he doesn't understand and I completely get that. From the outside this must be so bizarre. <u>NOTHING</u> *has happened. I'm making myself miserable by obsessing over a worry that isn't true.*

Even thinking the word in my head is ridiculous because I know *it not to be true. I just don't* believe *it and that's where C struggles to understand, and logically I get it, but you can't* <u>make</u> *yourself believe something. You can't logic away a belief.*

C asked why I thought this. Okay, here's my thinking:

1) I've had this happen before (in Stratford)
2) I don't know that I believe this is an illness – wouldn't a real child abuser think the same thing?
3) I feel weird around T. Why would a normal person see such vivid sexual and violent imagery around a baby and check if you had 'impulses'?
4) I feel wrong inside.

<u>Friday 2 April 2021 (11:13pm)</u>
Mood: Proud and hopeful
Positives today:
- *I ran over 7k!!!!*
- *I raised over £1,300 for NAS*
- *C & T*
- *Sunshine*

Today I ran over four miles and raised lots of money for a charity that's important to me. I'm really proud of myself – knowing where I was 8–9 weeks ago, I really challenged myself. Just this week I've run nearly twenty miles in training. It's been hard to have the motivation when you feel like shit/slept badly and it's scary to be so 'alone' with the thoughts on a run.

But I did it anyway.

And C & T were waiting for me at the finish line on a perfect spring afternoon and only my little family really knew what my achievement meant.

I listened to a podcast called OCD Stories and one woman's experience with POCD (paedophile OCD) after the birth of her baby. It was really helpful. I'm trying to think more of myself and not assume the worst about myself. I've really bonded with T this week. I'm giving him more of myself – bit by bit.

I only hold back because I don't want to hurt him.

Another podcast said, 'YOU CAN'T CONTROL THE THOUGHTS THAT COME INTO YOUR MIND. YOU CAN CONTROL THE ONES THAT STAY THERE.'

I'm not entirely sure what that means for me but it's useful to remember and also I'm so glad for other people telling their stories – I hope I can be that brave one day – it helps me to see that this is an illness, it's <u>not me</u>.

Intention for tomorrow: Be kind to yourself.

Monday 5 April 2021 (11:26pm)
Mood: Stronger
Positives today:
- Slept well
- Going to the park with all the kids
- Walk in the sunshine with Bob

I've had a great weekend, considering I'm still fighting my thoughts and feelings. But I've felt so much brighter and more level-headed. I'm using my CBT techniques and I'm proud of myself for pushing back. These thoughts are not a reflection of who I am. I'm trying to give myself a break.

Weirdly, in the last hour or so, I've spiralled slightly. I got cornered in the park earlier by a news crew and I ended up on the 10pm news. Only one person (my mother-in-law) texted me to say they saw me. I think being at the centre at a social media storm is a very real fear for me. Did I say something inappropriate? No. I answered Qs about going away on holiday this year. Will people be talking about me online? Possibly, if they recognise you're an actress. Will people be mean, say you're fat? Again, possibly, but that's okay. Are you fat?! You had a baby five months ago and ran 7k on Friday!! And it's not really about being fat – it's about no self-esteem and not feeling safe. Maybe something to discuss with E. Also, I find as soon as I get tired/stressed/worried, my intrusive thoughts about T come on really strong. The thoughts are not the problem – my reaction to them is. Take a breath. Challenge your thinking.

Intention for tomorrow: Ground yourself.

<u>Thursday 8 April 2021 (12:12am)</u>
Positives today:
- *Did a great event with NAS*
- *Lovely nap with T*
- *Seeing G & L*

I haven't written for a few days. I'm trying not to rely on this too much and sometimes I have a good day and am too knack-

ered to write. But I should write when things are going well – to read when they're not.

I hate when I think I'm getting better but then realise it's because I'm just resigned to the fact that I am a monster but I can live with it and keep it at bay. That's not true. Look at the evidence!!

You're not keeping yourself in check because one day you'll snap – you haven't, don't want to and definitely won't 'do' anything – so change your mindset.

The weather and the lack of focus this week (due to the 7k run) have made things tougher. The state of the house is getting me down, but it takes so much focus and energy to just get through the day and having functioned to care for T, I'm too exhausted to clean. Sometimes – a lot of the time – I don't see a point to it as I'm either trying to get better or truly am disgusting and evil, who cares about the fucking washing?

I am using my CBT skills – it's definitely helping. I felt this week that E seemed annoyed that I kept talking and going off on tangents, but that's probably just me.

I have to do something that I've always considered 'not an option for me' – so I'm going to do a painting and have a bath with T, even though I'm terrified.

Intention for tomorrow: Keep doing what you're doing!

Friday 9 April 2021

Positives today:
- Did a self-tape
- Sister-in-law's for a coffee
- Dad liked his birthday presents

Today has been a struggle – it feels like I've plateaued. I'm functioning, I can act normal and 80 per cent of the time not react to what's happening. But inside I'm dying a little every day. It's like death by a thousand cuts. Is this it for me now? Always going to have horrendous POCD intrusive thoughts? All day long? Whenever I'm near my baby? With therapy, exercise, medication and time, is this the best I'll get? It gives credence to it all being true because if it was a figment of my imagination, wouldn't it have worn off by now?

It's getting to the middle of the month, and my thoughts are getting darker – will this always happen around my period? I feel utterly trapped by own mind. I'm challenging my thoughts, changing my mindset, distracting myself, doing therapy and it's <u>just not lifting!</u>

I don't want to put C through any more. I just don't know what to do. It's so cruel. I think the world would be better without me and at least I could get some peace, but I can never leave as I wouldn't do that to everyone. We watched Palm Springs *with Andy Samberg on Netflix tonight and that's how it feels. Reliving the same nightmare of a day but sometimes I can let the thoughts pass and sometimes I can't. But the accumulative effect is that I'm utterly miserable.*

Intention for tomorrow: One more day.

<u>Monday 12 April 2021 (9:47pm)</u>
Mood: BLACK/DISGUSTED
Positives today:
- *Went for a run*
- *Had a shower*
- *Called the GP*

DEAR DIARY

*Had a really tough weekend. My hormones went crazy, and I totally lost it. Lost sight of everything I've been working towards. I can tell when something in the real world is making me mental and when its physiological. When it's hormones and chemicals in the driving seat. I became so hopeless and despondent at the weekend. I tried tapping into my CBT skills and better thinking, but I just couldn't access it. Everything became **V. BLACK.** I hate this feeling, this new reality I'm living. I've got a UTI, so my* thing *is hypersensitive which has doubled down on my thinking that I'm feeling something down there when I have these terrible thoughts. I become truly suicidal so quickly. I have some medication options, so we'll see.*

Things I'm frightened of:
1) *Bodily responses giving me 'evidence'*
2) *Becoming a child abuser.*
3) *Everyone finding out and disowning me*
4) *'Snapping' and doing something to hurt T*
5) *Being like this for the rest of my life*
6) *Never being able to fully enjoy watching T grow up*
7) *Feeling like dying is the only way out*
8) *Not being able to see that these thoughts about fearing child abuse are the illness. I'm not ill because I can't stand that it's true. I'm ill because I can't stop worrying about it*
9) *Doing something irreversible*
10) *C abandoning me*

I stopped writing in my journal here. Never wrote again. Never read it, until now.

Reading this back, my first thoughts are that I'm amazed by

how coherent it is. In my mind, I was a half-crazed, deranged woman madly scrawling nonsensical, asinine word-vomits that could and would be used against me in a court of law. But it's weirdly cogent and totally understandable. When writing this, I was lost in the dark. I thought this journal was the most incriminating piece of evidence and that I would eventually have to burn it for my own protection – certainly not publish for all to read.

But as scary as this is for me to put out there – and it's fucking terrifying – it's amazing what time and distance can do for your perspective. I would shake as I scribbled into this exercise book every night. I would defeatedly put it back on my bedside table, roll over and cry myself to sleep. Objectively, I can see writing it did help. It didn't feel like that at the time. I now also get a sense of where I swerved off onto an unhelpful track of thinking and where I righted myself. I can see that, as dead and numb as I felt, I was brimming with a love that I didn't know how to channel or understand and that I had turned it all into something creepy. I can see that it was someone desperately trying to break through a thick fog and get to the other side but who also wanted to leave something behind for her loved ones to read, if she didn't make it, so they would be able to understand.

I felt like I wasn't achieving anything day to day, but I was accomplishing the most astonishing feat of all: I was trying to get better while taking care of my son despite suffering this monumental brain malfunction.

Years on, seeing this woman's obvious contempt for herself and blatant sense of bewilderment, I have many reactions: I want to hug her, shake her, reassure her, bolster her, scold her.

But mainly I want to reach back and tell her it will be okay. That I know it doesn't feel like it, I know there's not even a glimmer of light on the horizon at the moment, but that she's not alone, she's not broken and she's not even that unusual.

I want to tell her when she's pregnant that the phrase 'intrusive thoughts' exists and to not be scared of it. I want to tell her that 70-100% of new mothers suffer with intrusive thoughts around harm coming to their baby (National Health Institute).[5] And 50 per cent will have unwanted thoughts about themselves harming their baby (NHI).[6] That because she has OCD, she wasn't able to let them go. I want to tell her that one in five mothers she knows will have suffered from a perinatal mental health illness. That it wasn't her fault that the blind faith she placed in the NHS was misplaced because of a lack of education and funding around these conditions, meaning that she was never going to win in that system. I want to tell her that her fixation with timelines and 'getting better' was born of the idea that 'postnatal' meant up to six months after birth. It doesn't.

When I was pregnant, all I saw were posters saying 'NEED HELP? JUST ASK.' My husband and I perversely joked that all of the mental health funding for women was spent on the posters and it's as if they never expected anyone to actually call. I did call. For nearly two years I called, but rarely was that call answered in any meaningful way. One day, I was sitting out on the steps in my in-laws' garden while they watched my baby for me, because I was too embarrassed to say I was phoning a helpline. I turned to PANDAS Foundation – they were engaged the six times I rang. That's why I've raised funds for them and Mothers Matter Cymru on Instagram. They are places that are largely donation-funded and they were so busy that day, I couldn't get through when I'd summoned up a scrap of courage to call in the first place.

I want to tell her that she has echolalia – that's why an earworm of a song or name would play over and over for forty-eight hours before fizzling out. Over and over and over and over and over and over and over and that this time, the safety of her child was at stake and that's why she couldn't simply 'let it go'. She's scanning for danger and risk-assessing and in her tired, scared, hormonal state, that perfectly normal instinct had gone haywire. That now, instead of an innocuous film quote or snippet of song, it's every terrible thing that can happen to a child in this world.

I want to tell her that in a few years, when she's better and just before she turns forty, she will be diagnosed with not only OCD but autism and ADHD. That there has always been a reason the world didn't quite make sense, and why her buzzy brain never stopped.

All the time I was writing this diary, I was looking for alternative treatments. I was just so desperate to get better. I looked into shock therapy. I researched magnetic treatments. I even remembered that Claire Danes's character in *Homeland* was on lithium. Would that help? Until finally, very much like in the book *We're Going on a Bear Hunt* that I would read to my little boy, I realised I couldn't go round it, I couldn't go under it, I had to go through it. I had to partake in the one form of therapy that I'd repeatedly read was the gold standard for OCD treatment.

What I truly needed, and couldn't start to recover until I'd spent my life savings on it, was CBT with a focus on Exposure Response Prevention (ERP).

ERP is a technique whereby you gradually expose yourself to your fears and learn to control your reaction and resist compulsions. This should be done initially with a trained therapist, and the key word is gradual. You start small, almost infinitesimal, and build up as you gain more control in seeing the ERP exercise through to the end, pushing through the anxiety spike – which would lead to your compulsion – and waiting it out until your distress passes. Sidenote: I didn't know how to spell 'infinitesimal' just now, so Word suggested 'infanticidal' – so that's a fun callback.

Back to ERP, which is not at all what I thought (session one: 'afraid of spiders? hold this spider'). I couldn't quite convince myself this could possibly work for me, as my obsessions and compulsions were largely invisible and mental. If I'd had a handwashing compulsion, I could physically sit on my hands and not do it. But how the hell are you supposed to stop a thought before you've thought it (you're not, by the way!) and how are you supposed to stop yourself from ruminating on it if thought processes are automatic (again, not what you're supposed to do)?

Nearly a year after I wrote these journal entries and I was still continuing to hurtle downhill, I found a place that I thought might be able to help me. The Maudsley Hospital in London is an NHS clinic that specialises in severe and complex cases of perinatal OCD. They offer a residential course of treatment: for two weeks you work intensively on Exposure Responsive Prevention with CBT. The criteria they required to be accepted were exacting and lengthy, and only applied to the most severe of cases. It seemed like a lifeline. I knew I had to try. My GP agreed I easily met the threshold and with a letter outlining my symptoms, history and medication/therapy to date from her and my new private OCD therapist, we applied to be considered. I even wrote personally to a specialist at the centre.

13 January 2022

Hello ▓,

I wrote to you a few months ago and thought I'd get back in touch. My OCD symptoms have become very acute and distressing. It's dominating my life. Every minute of every day for over a year now. I feel like I'm losing my mind.

I'm trying to get referred to you. My GP and therapist are on board but, as I'm based in Wales, there's a question of funding. I'm happy to fund the treatment myself and I can easily stay in London. However, my GP seems to think that I need to refer myself but with a letter from her?

I'm really quite desperate. I'm terrified of my own mind and I'm having regular panic attacks. It's been such a long time, I'm losing faith that I can get better. I have regular therapy, I'm on medication, I've done lots of reading on OCD but I keep getting worse.

Any pointers you could give me would be much appreciated.

Thank you for your time,
Kimberley x

DEAR DIARY

19 January 2022

Hi Kimberley

Sorry to hear that. Your GP needs to complete this attached form and then we can seek funding for an assessment and hopefully then treatment.

It's not possible to self-fund, I'm afraid, so try this first.

Let me know if you have any questions.

Best wishes

███ (Senior Administrator)

The form was comprehensive, to say the least. The markers I had to meet were incredibly high. I had to have completed two courses of therapy with no discernible progress (I had, paid for privately). I had to have tried two different medications to no avail (done and with deeply unpleasant side effects and withdrawals). I had to be considered severe enough of a case by my doctor to even apply (she was more than on board; I was rapidly declining before her eyes). We put all the information down and sent it off into the clinical ether.

After a nerve-wracking wait, they accepted my referral! I passed with flying colours; the only time in my nerdy life I had wanted to fail an exam. I qualified, and, if my health board would fund a two-week in-patient course of treatment, I could go. Hallelujah! A safe haven. A refuge where I wouldn't need to try to explain my condition, where I could speak freely and finally, finally, get the help I was desperately craving so I could move on with my life.

In amongst these letters, I was informed that the tenth anniversary of *Fresh Meat* was being celebrated at the BFI in London. There was a showing of an episode followed by a Q&A with us six main cast members alongside its creators Sam Bain and Jesse Armstrong. I went to London, trying to be normal, hoping for real life to snap back in. I love those five other guys so deeply – I had spent the best summers of my life with them – and we hadn't been all together in so long. It would be our first proper post-Covid event and it should have been a warm, friendly, joyous evening. And it was. These people make me laugh like no other but inside I crumbled at the thought they would all despise me if they knew what was really going on. I had the beginnings of a panic attack in my hotel room before heading to the lobby to meet them all before I chickened out. I managed to pull back from the cusp and within minutes of seeing and hugging them, we easily fell back into our absurd, giddy ways.

My husband checked in on me by text all evening. I was terrified that while on stage, I'd lose it – go off on a mental tangent, unable to repel the flurry of unwanted, intrusive thoughts or just the bone-deep sadness I'd been tamping down for over a year, where I'd start crying or clicking or shaking or smacking my head. People would either laugh or become disturbed. Cue government SWAT team or tabloid headline panic. However, I didn't – I sat and smiled. I loved seeing everyone again, including my agent, who I hadn't seen in the flesh since before getting pregnant! But every minute there was always the tap, tap, tap of OCD on my shoulder, trying to pull me under.

For the Maudsley Hospital, I arranged somewhere to stay. My

husband and son would even come with me, to be with me around my treatment as I didn't want to sever our bond or become too afraid to see them again. That's when I got a call from my local Primary Care Mental Health asking why I'd felt the need to apply to a specialist clinic. I explained we were nearly eighteen months on from the birth and I was steadily declining after jumping through every bureaucratic and tick-box hoop I'd been asked to. The man on the phone responded that there must be something they could do for me within my health board. They could offer me six weeks of phone therapy – not OCD-specialised, just general talking therapy but with someone with experience of dealing with OCD patients – and if I did that and still felt the need to go to the Maudsley, they would help with that.

Okay, I said. I was disappointed but understood and agreed to what I thought would be counterproductive and harmful therapy with yet another new person who knew nothing about my case. I was worried this would hinder the hard-won progress I'd made, but they agreed we'd chat again after the talking therapy course was complete and then we could proceed with funding my application for London.

A few weeks later, before I was due to start those empty, useless phone therapy calls, I received a letter from the Maudsley Hospital outlining that they were disappointed to hear that I wouldn't be taking up my place with them. They said that, as my health board had written to confirm they wouldn't be funding the treatment, they'd closed my file and good luck. That was it. I was going to jump through this six-week 'therapeutical' hoop for nothing while the Cwm Taf Morgannwg Health Board already knew that they'd terminated my application.

I asked again if I could self-fund. We were out of money, but we'd take out a loan. They told me no. I could apply again, but by the time I did, I'd be outside of the timeframe whereby they accept perinatal patients. Disheartened wasn't the word. I was devastated. It was as if not only were my local NHS mental health unit not helping me in any tangible manner, but it felt like they were actively trying to scupper any effort I made to get better. I knew, outside of my hazy, wrung-out mind, that wasn't their intention. It was just about the money. I *knew* that. But I *felt* so let down.

After much googling, a private clinic in London would take me. It was £350 for them to assess if I was eligible and then £7,000 pounds a week for their treatment programme, if I was successful.

I was so fucked.

7

All Aboard the Good Relationship

(Or This New Roommate is a Bit Needy)

I defy you to find a sturdier foundation for a relationship before starting a family than the one with my husband. You've probably spotted I don't use his name. Nothing ominous in it – I'm in the public eye, he's not. It didn't seem right to throw his details out there. Having said that, let's dig down into what happens when two human beings who love each other, create a third.

We had been together sixteen years when I gave birth. Sixteen whole years. We knew each other inside out (almost literally, after rigorously trying to conceive naturally for years). I knew what his opinion on something would be before he'd formed it himself and vice versa, and while I could be an enigma to others, he could read me like the proverbial book. A miniscule difference in tone and he'd ask, 'What's the matter?' when to everyone else around me, I seemed fine.

That would come up a lot over the next few years: 'You seem fine to me.' I was constantly being told by friends, family and strangers alike that I 'seemed fine' to them. Did they want me to 'perform' an OCD for them? Make them watch me wash my hands for two hours straight? That's not my subset. I've never had a problem with germs or contamination in that way. They could watch me sitting in a chair for hours, lost in my own mind. Spiralling down. Wheels within wheels. The trigger? An email. An offhand comment. Or postpartum, the unrelenting and brutal intrusion of highly disturbing thoughts and images.

There were certain aspects to becoming a mother that took me by surprise. For example, how much was I allowed to still be me? Wasn't it selfish to take time for myself to do things I enjoy? That wasn't really a problem, at that moment, as I couldn't quite seem to remember what I used to take pleasure in. I knew I walked a lot 'before'. With my dog, in the countryside. I read a lot too. Loved a good smutty, dark romance about a tattooed, muscled anti-hero and the sweet, innocent woman who makes him strive to be a better man. But those things felt wrong now. I couldn't disappear for a two-hour hike or lose myself in a book for hours like I used to. I had responsibilities, and the to-do list was never-ending. If baby clothes and bottles weren't washed and sterilised, the next cycle in a few hours' time would be a disaster, and I was already only hanging on by a thread.

That idea of 'sleep when the baby sleeps' would have been almost hilarious if I wasn't having a constant out-of-body experience. There are joke memes online, 'sleep when the baby sleeps, do the dishes when the baby does the dishes, mop when the baby mops, etc' which go some way to highlighting the absurdity of how I was supposed to manage my time now. It was relentless. The feeding – which could take up to two and a half hours, including winding, was still agonising. The changing, which – remove any OCD tendencies – was sometimes a two-man job. Weirdly, fluids didn't bother me. Any shade and consistency of baby poo didn't faze me, whereas my husband would gag while he held the baby's little feet up in the air so I could wipe.

But the sleeping? That was killer. When my son would nod off, he had to be held. Any attempt to put him down, so you could safely sleep too, was a complete non-starter. You know that scene at the beginning of *Raiders of the Lost Ark*, where Indy is sweating under the pressure of smoothly switching out the sacred idol with a bag of sand so as not to trigger any deadly boobytraps? It was a bit like that. I would think of that clip as I tried to lay him down in his crib, contorting my body to trick him into thinking he was still being held while attempting the Hug 'n' Roll from *Friends*. Hug for him, roll for me.

Once he was down and you'd crept away from him and he was STILL dozing happily, you'd look at the bombsite that was your living room. Or kitchen. Or bedroom. Or bathroom. As silently as a ninja, you'd collect used mugs and glasses. The plate with three-day old toast crusts lying abandoned on it. The muslins soaked in varying shades of semi-digested milk. You'd treat yourself to a wee. You'd do a leisurely, unhurried wipe because, why not? Spoil yourself. Doom scroll on your phone as an extravagance, all the while keeping one ear attuned to the slightest groan or gripe that may signal the baby needed you.

I would hear phantom crying quite a lot. You'd be pulling up your knickers with one hand, aimlessly looking at more successful people online and without thinking, reach out and press the flush automatically. Shit. Shit, shit, shit. Was that a whimper I just heard? You cock, you knobhead, you complete and utter shambles of a human being. You could have had half an hour of free time to do actual stuff but you've just ruined it. Just like you've ruined everything else. But then all would be quiet. Maybe you'd got away with it. You'd sigh heavily with a deep gratitude and go to get changed. Fresh pyjamas, how exciting. But you'd feel it before you heard it, the sucking in of air that signalled the howl about to explode from his tiny body. Resigned, you'd go and pick him up and start the feeding, changing, burping, soothing process once again.

This was so normal; I knew this. It was usual to struggle with a new role, a new life. I told myself over and over again every single person I knew who'd had a baby had felt the toll of those sleepless days and nights, the weight of responsibility to ensure the little one was getting everything they need. I saw my husband – bags under his eyes, two-day-old T-shirt – adjusting to our new normal. I felt all that too. But more pressing than any of that was this thick knot of dread snowballing in my gut telling me not to get too comfortable with having this new little guy around. It would end in tears, just you wait.

For one of us to wash up, or sleep undisturbed, the other had to have the baby. 'Can you have the baby?' became the cornerstone of your day. You'd start asking permission for the most basic things. 'Do you mind if I have a shower?', 'Is it okay if I try and get forty minutes' kip?', 'Do you want to watch the baby or do the washing?' For you to have any free time, your partner couldn't be with you, even if they were only a room away.

You'd lost your companion overnight. For months, we didn't spend any real time together and, as close as we were, this created a chasm that left both of us feeling slightly alone. And that was with a good, solid relationship. Throw in any other external relationship factors and it could become too much. I was still being honest with my husband about things not being right. I kept saying it and the less I took care of myself with fundamentals like sleep, eating healthily or brushing my teeth, the truer this became.

When my husband kept the baby downstairs for me to have a lie-down, I would almost run upstairs with relief. The fear that I was some paedophilic, serial-killing, blood-thirsty monster underpinned my every thought and action. I couldn't take the risk and slacken my awareness of every single thing I did, just in case. So going to the bedroom for two hours by myself was the closest thing I got to any sort of respite. Except I would lie in bed, curled into the tightest ball under the duvet and sob. My feet would be flexed and almost painful with how tense they were. I would constantly rub them together for comfort – something I would later discover to be an autistic trait called Cricket Feet, essentially a form of self-soothing.

I would finally pass out from exhaustion, but my sleep would be fitful and then I'd be roused from beneath the cloak of unconsciousness to hear the first step creak. The inescapable indicator that my husband was coming upstairs to give me the baby for a feed or because he was going to work and, with a soul-deep shame, my heart would sink. It would crush with fear and sadness that, once again, I must rejoin this waking nightmare. My chest felt like a submarine when it reaches Crush Depth. You know that video of a Coke can collapsing in on itself when pressure is applied? Like that. God, I was a terrible person. Why was I like this?

This continued for much of the first eighteen months.

Every time I came to, my mind would immediately check to see if it had all gone. The unknowable, yet relentless question of whether I was a monster. Like wearing a blanket of onyx treacle. I was being suffocated by OCD obsessions and compulsions. I would internally wince every time he cried, I would shake while cwtching him and I'd berate myself every moment of every day for not being better.

My husband was now essentially caring for two vulnerable people: his baby son and the shell of a human being that used to contain his wife. I went through the motions. I enjoyed nothing and even tiny glimmers of hope were immediately quashed with a 'how dare you enjoy that cute new smile he's doing?' I was a terrible person, rotten to the absolute core and my atonement was a never-ending loop of metaphorical self-flagellation. I was so fucking tired. Even with therapy, the wrong kind at first and eventually the right but very expensive kind, I was functioning better, but I wanted to go back to who I was *before*.

It would take me a very long time to grasp that this could never happen. But that wasn't actually the sealing of my fate I believed it to be. On the other side of this, there was a new me. A better me. Certainly, a stronger me. And a me that would alter from the inside out and learn more about my mad, wonderful brain than I could ever have expected. But right now? Right now, I hated my brain with an all-consuming intensity. It was trying to destroy me, and I feared it would win.

*

After six months, I knew I was *supposed* to want to be sexually active again, but the thought sent shivers down my spine. When you're trying to conceive, you have a lot of sex. And before getting pregnant, I'd hit a stride in my early thirties with a sexual confidence and not being afraid to lean into my sensuality and womanhood. It was incredibly liberating after a lifetime of self-doubt. But now, I genuinely believed that sex was never going to be an option for me again. Sex meant physical intimacy and allowing my mind to revel in fantasy. I couldn't allow myself to do that. What if we were mid-flow and thoughts of children or relatives or animals or death popped into my mind? Before orgasm, I would repeat the words 'don't think anything bad, don't think anything bad, don't think anything bad' in my mind. Of course, that's a self-fulfilling prophecy, so once the pleasure train had left the station, I'd be left reeling with the distrust that my sexual gratification was over the bad thing, not what I wanted or hoped.

Again, my husband was incredibly considerate. I didn't need to voice this as he'd already guessed. He was patient and said there was no rush – I'm going to bloody canonise him next – but he was still a human being who needed affection and intimacy and, well, naked time with his wife. And I'd be lying if I said that me pulling away from everything didn't affect our relationship. Just another department I was failing in, then.

After the birth, and for months after, I was obsessed with the idea of what was 'appropriate'. I was wildly confused by moving goalposts. Our bed was a real sticking point for me. Our bed, my favourite place in the world, traditionally my safe space if the world got a bit too big or loud in years gone by, was now a riddle. We tried to conceive in this bed. A lot. Now, our tiny baby was in the bed with us for feeds and soothing and I couldn't stop trying to figure out if that was okay. Can a baby be where sex has been? Ludicrous to you, I'm sure. But I couldn't solve this incessant problem that kept plaguing me.

The other facet I struggled with was that I was supposed to be two things at the same time now: a doting mother whose breasts were functional and wholesome, but also a wife and lover. Weren't boobs also meant to be sexy? I'm sure mine used to be? How would I know when to be which? What if I mixed them up? It confused me. Same with my vagina. What's okay? Things going in are sexual but things coming out, like babies or periods, are just part of the female experience. But what about tampons? Was that technically cheating? I should check. My exasperated husband reassured me that was nuts. He was probably right.

I'd always liked clear rules and distinctions. This is right, this is wrong. This is allowed, this is not allowed. I often mused while on family holidays why it was okay for us all to sit around a poolside table for lunch in bikinis but, if we were at home having dinner, I would never sit there in front of my in-laws in my underwear. What were the rules? And what had changed to change the rules? The weather, the country, the season, what?

But now I was overthinking everything, even down to choosing my knickers in the morning. Could I wear sexy underwear now I was a mum? I mean, I didn't really wear them before, so why was I considering it now? Did I want to wear sexy underwear? Why? In the end, I settled on some giant pregnancy pants that I wasn't ready to let go of no matter how far I moved away from being pregnant.

As much as my spiral down the postnatal helter skelter brought us closer together, in as much as I truly felt he was the only person whom even my paranoid, splintered mind could trust, there were hairline fractures cracking their way towards becoming a gulf. My only hope of reprieve had been this notion that in a very dark corner of my psyche, his hand was reaching out and grasping the one the 'shadowy Kim' was holding out for him. It kept me grounded as I lost all other points of contact with the familiar world around me. But that phantom grip could only stay strong for so long.

When I was pregnant, I remember reading a book about how I could have a positive birthing experience while sitting on the toilet and holding one arm above my head. They claimed this would give you an idea of the stamina you would need throughout contractions and that by using your breath, you could take control back. A Gaian image of me squatting in crystal-clear waters in an ancient rainforest and birthing my own baby, no drugs, no interventions, the only sound, birdsong, soon fizzled when my arms began to shake with the effort of it. And I was only practising on the loo. Well, both our reaching arms were beginning to shake with the toll this condition was taking on us.

My only objective was to make it through. In the early days, I would stare at the kitchen clock on our wall, telling me it was 11:51 and convince myself I just had to make it to midday. That's all. Nine minutes. Try not to think or feel or do anything except stare at the second hand winging its way around and wait for midday. When, inevitably, it hit the head of the hour, I would feel no relief or sense of accomplishment, and would then push myself to make it to quarter past. And so on. It went on like this for weeks. I would feed him, change him, bathe him, rock him, read to him, take him out where Covid permitted, but always have one eye on the clock. Eventually it moved from minutes to hours and about a year and a half in, I could maybe manage a shift of four hours without needing to clock-watch. There was no time for anything – or anyone – else; I had to trust our relationship would weather this storm because I didn't have a molecule of energy to spare on it.

★

Other relationships in my life suffered tremendously as well. Jess, the Jess I could tell anything to, wouldn't be able to handle the intensity, absurdity and brutality of this . . . this *thing* I had become, I told myself. I was ashamed and terrified to confess it all to her. I pulled back, then withdrew. I stopped all social interactions and replied to texts sparsely, just letting her know I was postnatally 'unwell'. I wouldn't find out for years to come that one day, when Jess dropped a Costa coffee off on the doorstep as a treat, she met the health visitor on her way out. 'Are you going in?' she asked. Jess immediately promised that she wasn't breaking any Covid regulations, just leaving a coffee for me outside. Apparently, she gave Jess a knowing look, glanced back at the house, then said, 'You should go in.' Same with my dad – he had to stop asking me how I was as I made very little eye contact and just mumbled platitudes. He ended up having to check in with his son-in-law for a more truthful update instead.

Meanwhile, my husband continued to try to keep things light and as normal as possible. He decided to paint our utility room (I know – get us!) and he tried to engage me in picking the colour. I vividly remember not having a single view on it. Nothing, not an iota of an opinion, zipped through me at all. I didn't have time for walls; I was battling an invisible war just to make it through to tomorrow. Paint? What the hell was he talking about? I was bewildered and mumbled a 'whatever you like'. Quite frankly, my dear, I didn't give a shit.

That was a huge red flag. We always argued about paint colours. Our first home, a tiny, terraced miner's house in the South Wales

Valleys, needed completely gutting – literally taking back to the brick. Apart from the hugely specialised jobs – it didn't have any central heating, for example – we did everything ourselves. We sanded every skirting board, gave every inch two or three coats of paint and chose every detail together. When realising that most of the house had quite an earthy palette, we briefly decided to try and be a different, cooler couple and bravely paint one wall in the tiny spare room a bright crimson colour. It was ten to five in the afternoon and, within three strokes, we realised it looked terrible, it wasn't us and promptly raced back to B&Q to change it before they closed.

Our second and current home was us moving up the property ladder. More bedrooms for all those rosy-cheeked, golden-haired children we were bound to have. An old Victorian house, again needing a full renovation, which we tried to restore to its former glory. We bickered about every shade of green, every type of kitchen cupboard and every placement of vintage film poster or framed memory. We cared so much because it felt important. We were making this house into a home for our future family. But now, as I stared at the deep teal paint he was about to apply to the wall, I couldn't have given a flying fuck. He could have done a Nineties-Changing-Rooms-leopard-print-and-scarlet-brothel theme and as long as I could get to the washing machine to deal with the endless piles of babygrows, it meant nothing to me.

Same with cleaning. If it didn't pertain to the baby and his hygiene, it didn't exist to me. I washed and sterilised bottles and dummies meticulously; he always had a freshly laundered onesie to wear. Fluffy hooded towels awaited him after his bath and his cot had a hotel-level turnover of valeted sheets and blankets. But I couldn't have told you the last time I washed my face or brushed my hair. Showers were a luxury someone as disgusting as me didn't deserve and I just didn't see the point. All my energy was poured into caring for my son and fighting to the death with my OCD.

And in this scenario, romance does not thrive.

As I became more accustomed to the status quo, I pulled away from everything. Including my husband. It frightened me to discover that he couldn't help me this time. I felt no comfort or relief in my safest of places. He wasn't able to slay this big black, shape-shifting dragon like a white knight, so the only person I could rely on was myself. And as I currently couldn't trust myself, I was basically fucked. If I'm being brutally honest, I just wanted someone to take this all away. Feminism be damned in this ferocious battle for dominance over my own mind. But another little piece of my heart cracked at the knowledge that, even if I was a damsel in distress, no medical personnel or even the great love of my life could save me. The sadness made me curl in on myself. When I did make some headway in recovery, I felt this unintentional drive to never, ever be that vulnerable again. Nobody could help me but me. I wouldn't make the mistake of placing my trust in anyone ever again. It was too painful when you were inevitably left to drown alone.

At one point my husband couldn't take not *doing* something anymore and bundled us all into the car on a frozen but sunny day and drove us to the beach. Something stirred in the back of my mind that he must be desperate. He hates the beach in winter, finds it melancholy and too contemplative. I love the beach and always suggest we go; he always moans. This must be bad. He'd been reading up on cold-water swimming and it potentially being beneficial to your mental health. He's not the black-and-white thinker; it's me that usually has a 'one dip and I'll be cured' mentality but I could see he was all out of ideas and had to try *something*.

I was in my bathers under my clothes and winter coat, and when we arrived around sunset, it truly was sublimely beautiful. Epic cliffs, roaring waves and a golden syrupy glow was cast low along the sand. It meant nothing to me. I was devoid of feeling. He had the baby bundled up in layers and strapped to his chest, the dog was on the lead barking his head off and he realised he'd timed this wrong, as the tide was about half a mile out. We stood next to some rockpools, and he said I should strip and get in. I did. I took off my clothes, no questions asked, and proceeded to squat in an icy puddle of water. The only part of me that was getting any cold-water therapy was my minge. The cold centred on that one area did distract me from my intrusive thoughts, obsessions and depressive state for a short while, so evidence it could work.

While crouching in a ball, my arsehole, cooch and feet the only parts of me submerged, I blinked up at my husband, who, wrapped up in his coat and hat, our baby enveloped in a snowsuit held to his chest, and a powerful beast on a leash at his side, did have an air of the white knight but he'd met his match this time. A silent 'what now?' passed between us. A passerby stopped to ask if I was a wild swimmer. Wild swimmer? Read the room, love. I'm squatting in a tiny pool of glacial water that doesn't reach past my ankles, in the bleak midwinter, trying not to cry and clearly in the middle of a full-blown nervous breakdown. What about this scene makes you think I'm ripe for recruiting to your wild swimming club, which meets just over there by the rocks, every Monday?

'Thanks, I'll think about it,' I told her. She happily chatted away for the next few minutes, my husband keeping a side eye on me to ensure I was still holding on.

When she cheerily waved goodbye, he said we should go and handed me a towel and thick coat. I'd disappointed him again. He'd tried to fix me and I was just not fixable. He said he was sorry; he thought it might help. I told him it did. As we headed off the sand, I spied and scooped up a pleasingly smooth-looking pebble: pale grey with a thin streak of white calcite. I'd been reading somewhere on the internet at some godforsaken hour about using natural objects, like rocks, to ground you. When you start to spiral or feel disconnected from the world, you can use the touch and feel of the Grounding Stone to calm you and keep you in the present. It's something solid and real to focus on. There are some that say there are earthly properties and spiritual elements that heal you but as there's next to no science to back that up, I find it about as beneficial as someone telling me I'm a 'typical Libra'. In other words, fucking useless. But just like the lemon in my pocket for morning sickness, there was a certain comfort in holding something tangible in the palm of my hand when my head was all cotton wool and nightmares. And what did I know? Maybe it would connect me to the stability of the earth's energy and cure me. My husband looked back and asked what I'd picked up. 'Magic rock,' I mumbled.

We got back in the car and drove home. I sat in the back, ostensibly so I could be nearer the baby if he needed anything, but also partly because it was easier to soundlessly cry back there without drawing too much attention. My husband was a silent, defeated chauffeur no longer sure how to reach his wife.

★

I've since learned through my OCD therapy that him giving me reassurance is a way of, unknowingly, perpetuating the problem. He will never be able to reassure me enough; I will always go back for another fix. So, we keenly started to practise 1) me not asking if I was a monster, a murderer, a child abuser, a terrible person, a psychopath, beyond redemption and 2) him not telling me it was all okay, that he'd known me for twenty years, I wasn't any of those things and if I could just see myself how he sees me . . . It was arduous and painful, like breaking any habit. But whereas with giving up smoking, when you *know* it's for the best in the long run, this just felt unnecessarily cruel on top of an already horrible situation. Having said that, within six to eight weeks of doing this, we really began to see a difference. I was standing on my own two feet, having to tell myself I didn't need that certainty. I was becoming more self-sufficient and gained a control over my recovery. I was getting stronger and less emotionally distressed.

As I slowly improved over the next couple of years, I convinced myself it was because I could rely on myself to understand when my brain got sticky and obsessively spiralled and what to do when it happened. I couldn't be blindsided like that again. If and when I plummeted backwards, I would be ready. The side effect of this was me pulling away from the relationship, and my husband pulling away because he thought that's what I wanted or needed. Communication got less frequent and, in that void, we developed an increasingly tenuous link to each other. We were growing distant. We could both feel it. But that felt so secondary to me getting better, it was easy to put it on the back burner for a year or two. Until that chasm became the main story.

SHE SEEMS FINE TO ME

When you go through something life-changing, it really shouldn't come as a shock to you that your life changes. But it does. Fundamentally. Utterly. And you must change with the times. You have to or you won't survive it. You adapt to each 'new normal'. Each new phase of childhood for your child and each new unlocked horror of the illness for you. Life moves on, your baby grows but you feel ever more stuck as you try to keep up. Like doing the Macarena submerged in treacle. This pretty much happens to everyone who has a baby; your life is just different in a thousand small ways now. If you're in a relationship, you both change when you become parents as you have new roles: carer, disciplinarian, teacher, playmate, the master of twenty decisions an hour. Are they allowed peanut butter yet? Should I just give them the thing they're crying over or hold out to use this as a teachable moment? Does this ham look okay to you? How long can a nappy legally be left on for if you've run out? Do you know where their shoes are? Coat is? Bag? Dummy? Book? Blanket? Wipes? Spider-Man?

It was a noisy and busy time. All the time. Now imagine you have all that plus the tap, tap, tapping on your shoulder of OCD. *I must remember to check my heartrate when he's sucking his dummy, or did I do his car seat up properly or accidentally-on-purpose leave it undone? Have I hit him in the last five minutes but forgot because I was making him this sandwich? Did he die in the thirty seconds it took the kettle to boil? What if I pour boiling water all over him? I don't want to, but I'm really knackered and can't think straight, and I might just do it in a moment of madness and then it's ruined.*

To my husband, from the outside nothing had happened to

cause me to be standing in the middle of the kitchen crying, but for me it was a never-ending diatribe, and I was one mouldy slice of bread from losing it. We started snapping at each other because we were sick and tired of trying to explain how we felt. Resentment, distance and rejection began to spread like invisible mycelium until our connection eventually bore an ugly, fungal fruit.

We argued more or went days without speaking. Two to three years of caring for a child, while one of us was dealing with the ongoing crush of a mental health condition so misunderstood that even experts were looking to me for answers, had left its mark. Then my husband started developing mental health issues of his own as a result of the incredible toll the whole ordeal had taken on him. He was drained and worn out at being the 'strong' one and we started to have less and less we could be bothered to talk about. The intimacy of starting a family together had been swamped by day after day of the unseen push against the system, or nature, or each other, and hadn't it all just been easier before?

Yes and no. It's so tempting to retrospectively romanticise the past. One more significant marker in my recovery was seeing things how they were, not how I wished or dreaded them to be. The past was a mish-mash of ups and downs, brutal blows and dizzying highs. The future would almost certainly be the same. The present was all I had and I could only tackle it a moment at a time.

★

Somewhere in amongst all this, I decided to grab the bull by the balls, or whatever the saying is, and took part in Welsh channel S4C's show *Iaith ar Daith* (Language on a Journey).

SHE SEEMS FINE TO ME

You take one well-known Welsh person who can't speak Welsh, pair them with another well-known one who can and send them off on a road trip to discover Wales and the language. I was paired up with the lovely, joyful Matthew Gravelle. I had never worked with Matthew professionally but had known him personally through his wife, Mali Harries, for ten years. We shot a medical drama called *Critical* back in 2014 and, as the two Welsh ones, drove back and forth from Cardiff to Longcross Studios in Surrey for the best part of a year. Mali came to my wedding that December and one of my abiding memories of my Big Day is coming out to greet everyone after the nuptials and Mal having one foot up on a table painting her toenails because she'd forgotten to earlier. It was a good tone-setter for the rest of the day, and we had the most wonderful time with dancing, laughter and of course, Christmas trees dotted everywhere. And all our tables were named after famous TV/film detectives. I'm nothing if not consistent.

Matthew and I set off for a week of filming where I had to learn and speak Welsh. It was terrifying but taught me two very important lessons about recovery and giving myself permission. Firstly, that I was allowed to focus on something else. That week, when I had to concentrate on trying to translate everything in my head from the English to my most available Welsh didn't leave room for other intrusive thoughts to make much headway. And secondly, and probably most importantly for me, it was okay to make mistakes. Giving a sentence a go in rudimentary Welsh was better than not trying at all. The more I failed, the better I became. I remembered the tense or verb I used last time was wrong, so corrected it on my next attempt. And every time I sounded like an idiot or talked utter nonsense (for instance, I mixed up the words for 'ice' and 'sex', although in my defence, the words are 'rhew' and 'rhyw', like the word 'rue' with a rolled 'r'), I would overcome the embarrassment and notice that the world didn't end. I repeatedly told Matthew I was very excited about our upcoming afternoon doing contrast water therapy at Fire and Sex. But once I was past feeling foolish in this whole endeavour, I lost my hesitancy to push through and try again. My brain began to flex in a way it hadn't before and soon I was speaking more fluent Welsh.

And that was exactly what I needed in my recovery, with regard to being frank, open and honest about what true OCD was. My thinking had always been that I could never share with anyone that I was unwell because of the content of my intrusive thoughts. It took me so long to truly realise that the content never mattered; my obsessive need to analyse, fix and neutralise did. So, I worked on that part instead and I started to get better because I had a clearer head, not a permanently foggy one, which is OCD's preferred environment. If I fell into the trap of doing a compulsion (like tapping my head, clicking my fingers, ruminating, body checking) it wasn't the end of the world; I could just try again next time. Trying to curate your thoughts perfectly, neatly labelling and storing them in boxes, is a thankless, and frankly futile, task. It's like trying to file and catalogue dust. It's exhausting and ultimately pointless.

Although I'd always been a very tactile person with people I was comfortable with, I found that I'd stopped even basic touch with everyone, including my husband. I didn't hug him, snuggle up to him, hold his hand or kiss him anymore and he didn't push me by initiating it. It was like I was contaminated, and I wanted to touch as few things as possible to keep the infection from spreading. Ironically, it didn't happen with my baby because I'd always pushed through in that respect. I knew if I didn't pick him up out of fear – just once – I would never go back. But I took my eye off the ball with my husband, complacency duping me into thinking that we would always be solid. I knew it had become a problem when, for the first time in nearly twenty years, I didn't hold his hand on take-off during a flight. I saw him turn a shade paler, but I just didn't know if I could or should reach out. I was guarded, and it had become habit. When I realised this, I slowly started to reach out for my husband more, not fighting the instinct that I shouldn't as it could taint him; as if the repulsive nature of my OCD-thinking could physically pollute him too. And this was an intolerable existence I wouldn't wish on anyone, *especially* not him.

*

Now, years later, I think what this saga took from us was that he was the person who knew the very heart of me, even when I didn't, but could no longer reach me in the same way. We've been rebuilding it and we're stronger in completely different ways now too. This will eventually become another chapter in our story. We silently fight for each other every day and it's still true that I want nothing more than for him to be the first person I tell about something funny I just saw, or a new bit of local gossip or that I didn't get that job I really wanted. He's there. Every. Single. Time. Just as I am for him. And as for the physical, romantic side of things, we're back to where we were pre-baby. Alright, maybe my boobs are a bit saggier and he's a

ALL ABOARD THE GOOD RELATIONSHIP

shade greyer, but I unlearnt what I thought OCD needed to teach me. Bit by bit, moment by moment, until years later that's your new habit. I feel like I've reclaimed my body, with every glorious bump, lump and stretchmark a badge of honour. When you're with somebody for over twenty years, your bodies change. We've fallen in love time and again with each corporeal incarnation of each other.

It seems we've always been waiting in the wings for each other. Cheering the other on.

Your wedding day isn't your rom-com finale. Showing up every day, until the final curtain, is.

8

Who Do You Think You Are?

(Some Kind of Superstar?)

When you've been out of work for a while, it can be really difficult to get back in the game. People want new and fresh. Hell, I knew this even when I *was* new and fresh. Unless the perfect part comes along at just the right time, a lot of actresses in their late thirties/early forties – especially those from a regional/working class background – will be the 'Mum', the 'Wife', the 'Female Colleague' or the 'Sister'. Someone younger or much more famous is the 'Love Interest', and actors with better connections than you could *ever* hope to have, simply get into the rooms you need to be in to even be considered for the part. And there are some rooms you won't ever even know exist. They're not for you. There is no regional room at this Upper-Class Inn, so to speak. But feel free to pop yourself and your not-London-based Donkey down to the Bit-Part Stable.

Of course, as an actress, there are things that you can do to help your career. Namely going to private school, coming from a wealthy family, having a close relation/family friend already in the business, and not growing fatter, uglier or older. Okay, no one quite manages the last one, though they try, but the point is that I didn't have any of those things. I learnt that you could graft away, make solid contacts and produce good work, but without those family funds to fall back on or knowing the 'right' people, you'd always be toiling away with one hand tied behind your back.

However, I do think this is changing. I think there are more working/lower middle-class people from outside of the industry pushing through. It's not an imperative to live in London like it was. And body positivity and a better understanding of neurodiversity are all moving in the right direction. But for most of my career, you couldn't be even slightly overweight, weird or difficult to work with unless you were also rich and connected. That's life.

I went back to work about ten months after my son was born. I was filming *The Tuckers*, and bizarrely, the best acting of my career was done trying to come across as normal to my colleagues. I found the only break from the daily barrage of psychological terror were the moments between 'action' and 'cut' where there was silence on set, and I had to be someone else for a few, glorious moments. Knowing what they were going to say, how they felt and what they thought about their current state of affairs was incredibly freeing. There was a relief in that space. On 'cut!', the reality of my situation would flood back in, and I would be reminded to put my nose to the compulsion grindstone. If I wasn't on watch, then who would be? Sometimes the only way I got through a take was the knowledge that I had a hundred witnesses to where I was and what I was doing, and my baby was safely on the other side of the valley. A literal mountain of protection.

WHO DO YOU THINK YOU ARE?

Filming and simply *doing* my job was a kind of muscle memory for me; I remembered this version of myself. I used to do this before I'd given birth and lost my mind, and I could do it again. I didn't fool myself into thinking I could be a working mother who 'had it all'; I was perfectly happy with my baby being safe, some money coming in and making it to the end of the day before I collapsed into a melancholic heap of exhausted heartache when I got home. I would barely sleep all night while my brain played out terrible, terrible things in my mind. I'd nod off around 4am and my alarm would go off at 5.30am for my 6am pick-up. I lived like this for about three months, so while being back out in the world definitely helped some, it also set me back because I was living an unsustainable lifestyle.

Still, acting was my escape route. Every day I was being given permission to not be myself. My make-up calls were long, so it would just be me and the make-up artist, Mica, who became a great friend. We would listen to Lionel Richie (her favourite) and drink coffee (my favourite) and sometimes, if the baby had been up all night, she would encourage me to nap while she did my make-up. I had blonde hair extensions, false nails, fake tan, fake eyelashes, layers and layers of foundation and lip gloss. It almost became like a suit of armour for me.

There was one scene where I had to be upset and vulnerable with another character, but I couldn't quite tap into it. Ironic, I know. As the cameras turned over and I waited for the sound team to announce they were 'speeding' and the first assistant director to declare 'Action!', I let a small crack prise itself open within me to allow my real emotions and the character's to bleed into each other. Like when you pour thick kids' paint into another colour, but you haven't mixed them together yet.

They are separate but can never be separated; it creates this fascinating marble effect. The one colour snaking a new path through the other, creating something new, something beautiful. I thought about how I'd so severely let my son down, but what it resulted in was the character's reaction rather than my own. She was flighty and fun-loving but determined to have her own way. Suddenly I was seeing my own situation through another character's lens and it didn't quite hold up to scrutiny. What a waste of time. She wouldn't stand for this nonsense. She didn't get it. But in the end, she found me so pathetic, it felt like she was crying for me rather than the other way around.

I got a new job on a big TV production, *The Baby*. The irony of the title of the show wasn't lost on me, nor was the fact that I had to spend all of my time acting the part of a competent, judgemental mother. There were babies everywhere on set and what should have occurred to me was that I didn't have worries or intrusive thoughts around them. But it didn't because logic had no place in this new world order.

I had to travel to London and stay in a hotel for a few days while I was filming. It was a strange mix of missing my little boy and being relieved I could stand down for forty-eight hours. The car ride from Paddington Station to the hotel was interminable. I was trembling in the back seat, desperately listening to a podcast by an OCD expert, attempting to implement what they were saying in real time. But everything was just out of reach for me. I barely made it through check-in, tumbling into my room with my suitcase before I had a full-blown panic attack. I couldn't breathe, there were invisible hands at my throat choking me and I was bent over trying to get a hold of myself. I was continuing with Zoom therapy with the nice lady. I was on medication. Nothing was working! I didn't want to call my husband, as he'd already got enough going on looking after the baby by himself, and none of my friends knew enough of the backstory to phone them. Not even Jess. I felt a loneliness so dominant that I literally fell to my knees before slumping forward onto the floor. I lay on my front and stared at the carpet fibres. I had to go to work tomorrow. I had to be professional. This earthquake was shattering the world around me and nobody else felt even the slightest tremor.

I made it through filming and came home. The earth spun and the sun rose but there was nothing but *this*. This pestilence of the mind. Jobs came and went. I got better at masking and hiding but worse at connecting or engaging. My agent and his assistant were incredible throughout this period, but eventually I just knew they'd need to give up on me too but I was too exhausted to care. I'd come a long way from the sensitive little actress whose heart was broken when she was made to feel too fat or ugly. Sadly, it wasn't the liberating feeling my twenty-something year-old self had hoped it would be.

I'd fought the world, and the world won.

★

Admittedly, there are one or two choices I could have made that would have certainly helped me to get back into work. I could have stayed the same size as I was at twenty-one (which I was repeatedly told was too big even then). I recall leaving the costume fitting for *Wild Child* in tears as they'd been sent a rail of 'sample size' (read: size zero) designer clothes and even as a slinky size 8, I had boobs and hips (remember I was nearly 21 playing 16). I was told that they 'didn't know what to do with me'. I remember feeling humiliated and just so confused.

I didn't *feel* fat and, in fact, I had always been told I was 'too skinny'. I hadn't changed in appearance since the audition process when I'd got the job. I was later pulled aside and told that maybe I was 'enjoying the set catering a bit too much' over on *Cranford*. Again, I was confused. I was working 14–15-hour days on both productions. I wasn't eating more than anyone else. How was I supposed to stay nourished and have the stamina to get through months of long shoot days in a healthy way? I realise now I just answered my own question. Health had nothing to do with it. Over the years I would watch actresses literally survive on a pure liquid diet instead of actual food (a mix of water, lemon juice, maple syrup and cayenne pepper) or grazing from a Tupperware of, essentially, bird seed in between takes in order to keep their weight down.

I could have moved to London and gone to the right parties, had famous partners, not been weird. I could have been less honest about how I was finding motherhood; I could have got some Yummy Mummy photoshoots and collaborations with magazines and baby clothing companies instead. I could have subsisted on water and seeds too and then posted pictures of myself online biting into a giant, greasy burger, so you'd think that I was just naturally thin, and *you* – the couch-sitting doom-scroller were the odd one out for not being able to maintain a miniscule frame living on junk food. I could have worn more make-up, or less make-up, or dressed provocatively for 'likes' or fashionably for kudos. I could have taken out loans to have my teeth done, boobs done, endless skin peels and weight-loss injections. And then maintain it, indefinitely. I could have chosen not to share the scariest, darkest time in my life on Instagram. But that is exactly what I did.

WHO DO YOU THINK YOU ARE?

I'd been persuaded to join Instagram by other actors on *The Tuckers* when my son was around ten months old. Wasn't it all just photos of posh lunches and Botox and unaffordable holidays in Dubai? Yes, but I'd get free dungarees.

I'd do it.

I created an account and waited for Big Dunga to reach out and then I could write #AD underneath a perfectly curated and filtered picture of me – just like a real actress. But within a couple of months, I realised it wasn't for me. I had a choice: conform and feel constantly inadequate, or make it something else, my own. I kept thinking of something my husband said to me once, when all this started, and I tearfully asked him, 'Why is it so easy for everyone else?'

'What do you mean by that, Kim?'

'Just everywhere you look, other women are just getting on with it.'

'Where are you looking?'

'Well, social media, I guess.'

'Kim, if someone saw your Facebook, they would think you're loving it and "just getting on with it" too.'

That stopped me in my tracks. Was I adding to the fakeness and heaping inadequacy onto someone else? My mind fled back to that smiling picture of me with my new baby and realised no one would have guessed I cried for an hour straight afterwards.

I dabbled in being more honest and waited for the backlash. It never came. The more frank I was about motherhood and mental health, the more people reached out to me with nothing but compassion and consideration, sharing their stories with me and slowly bringing postnatal OCD out of the shadows, where it thrives like a woodlouse (or Granny Grey as we call them in South Wales).

The more positive the response, the bolder I became. I gained confidence and a sense of purpose. I may have to live this reality for the rest of my days but maybe there were others out there? If I didn't survive this, maybe I could be that voice that someone would find in some godforsaken corner of the internet in a desperate midnight googling session, frantically searching for talk of perinatal symptoms that didn't align with just depression or anxiety. That would be nice. It gave me a brief but needed glimmer of light.

Being 'vocal' about my mental health was a huge part of my recovery, even if pre-baby me would have derided me being more open about it. Don't get me wrong, I still frequently shit myself that I've made a terrible mistake after posting something a bit more real than 'Avocado on toast with my bestie!' or 'Mama's going OUT-out!', which I am certainly guilty of. I often wonder if I've just irrevocably exposed myself in a way that will ruin my career or permanently alter how people see me, but it's been the best practice for the 'maybe but that's okay' method I've ever done. I regularly brace myself for the Beauty and the Beast-style pitchforked lynch mobs and wait for social services or the police to knock on my door. My OCD still goes crazy, internally yelling RETRACT! RETRACT! RETRACT! BEFORE YOU RUIN EVERYTHING!

But posting on Instagram didn't ruin anything. In fact, it opened up my heart again to the world not being such a cruel and terrible place. Over the years, I've had thousands of messages, and I think they can most aptly be summed up into one simple sentiment: 'I thought it was just me.' I've received messages from mothers whose children are now in their twenties or thirties saying, 'I'm crying because this was me all those years ago and I was too scared to tell anyone.' I've had husbands and partners tell me that they recognise this in their loved ones and see it more clearly now. But the absolute best messages I've had are from new mums who tell me that they've not been coping, they've never seen anyone speak about these symptoms and, feeling less alone, they've called their doctor to make an appointment. Maybe I wasn't a medical marvel, a freak or a write-off; there were others out there who were suffering in silence. Hopefully by starting this discussion on a public forum, I'd helped their recovery time become a fraction of mine.

I work in an industry that's image-based and fuelled by comparison. You're judged on how thin and beautiful you are, who you're sleeping with and who you know. Every other actor looks to be working while you languish in unemployment and unproductivity. But the older and more experienced you get, the more you see the hidden tells of bullshit. Someone might be all over Instagram promoting a new show, but the truth is they filmed it two years ago and haven't worked since. Or, my personal favourite, an actor posts a wonderful series of intense, actor-y shots in ludicrous poses in a shirt that's too big for them or holding a vintage phone in their hand, thanking a bunch of people for putting them on the cover of a magazine you've literally never heard of and wouldn't know where to buy, to discover they paid thousands of their own money to some PR company to set all this up.

As an actress, the idea of being a success was always at the forefront of my mind. For me, failing meant ruin. Ruin meant being alone. Of course, some of this was because a lot of my upbringing seemed to teach me that success was based on the premise of being a good girl: work hard, don't make a fuss, go above and beyond to be helpful and useful, and therein lies your worth. And so giving birth a few weeks after my thirty-sixth birthday, I thought I knew myself and my limits. I'd been through a lot in my life and overcome it. Professionally, I'd recovered from plenty of failures – like the time I spilled coffee down the especially requested white dress right before a big audition, or when I threw up outside a casting director's house because that slightly out-of-date egg and cress sandwich had upset my stomach. Or when I got too hot and slowly removed my cardigan and joked, 'I'm not trying to seduce you for the part,' before I swiftly pulled the woolly garment back over my shoulders when no one in the room laughed.

But I'd lost myself so profoundly in that fourth trimester that it was as if I was a smashed vase that had been glued back together all wrong. The pieces were all there but in the wrong place and the more I tried to fix it, the worse it became. I felt fragmented and scared and sad – so unbelievably sad – when I didn't feel I had any right to be. Some women couldn't get pregnant at all, some women lost their babies, some women had nothing and no one. The guilt was devouring me whole. It's easy to sit here now and look back at my postnatal self and see objectively that I was being too hard on myself. Of course everything was a learning curve, but back then, probably due to hormones, chemicals and environmental factors, I couldn't breathe with the stifling self-scrutiny.

Mental health conditions thrive in the dark. The more you keep them to yourself, the more confirmation bias you will find everywhere you look that those gloomy and sinister thoughts were right all along. The more isolated you are, the more ripe you are for the picking. There's also a trick OCD likes to play to halt your recovery by whispering, 'But people don't know the real you.' You can function day to day, go to work, care for your kids, meet up with friends but really, it's all a façade, because they don't know the REAL you. You're keeping that hidden, out of shame or fear, and that always gives your OCD a 'yeah, but . . .' to fall back on. My family loves me. *Yeah, but they don't know my darkest thoughts.* I'm good at my job. *Yeah, but if everyone found out, that would be taken away.* I'm a good mother. *Yeah, but only because you do your compulsions and monitor everything you do.* For me, Instagram got rid of that inexorable '*yeah, but . . .*' because I'd told strangers all over the world the worst parts of my life and I still got unbelievably kind-hearted and empathetic engagement. Either it resonated with someone, or those who had no experience of it were caringly curious. Shining a light on those darker, less talked about symptoms, those taboo, terrifying and daunting ones, forced my OCD to confront a lot of holes in its narrative.

Are there horrible messages? Yes – but rarely. And they're good practice, too. The world keeps spinning, people I love still love me back, and my little boy is happy and glad I'm his mum. It's like confronting the bully and *them* having to shrivel under the scrutiny instead of it constantly being you. By being open about my struggle, the tables have turned, and it only makes me braver and more determined to not live another moment of my life inauthentically – virtually or in reality.

Posting about OCD on Instagram was one of the scariest things I've ever shared with the world. Sometimes I'm still mortified that people will read it and look at me differently. I didn't have to share this. I could have pretended it didn't happen, but I couldn't do that to those who were still drowning behind me, just because I'd finally reached the albeit still-damp sands of land.

Maybe posting on Instagram was the best 'fuck you' to OCD I've ever done.

One of the strange, wonderful and incongruous juxtapositions to all of this on social media was that one day, the International Day of Happiness 2024 to be exact, I thought I would inject some silliness into proceedings and asked people to send me their crappiest Dad jokes. I love a pun or a stupid play on words, it's always made me chuckle, so I blind-read jokes on camera and laughed.

This blew up in a way I could never have predicted. The first video has been viewed over 1.4 million times. People flocked to my account. My followers increased by the tens of thousands and I eventually found that these videos could raise money for charity too. I received messages from people of all ages, all over the globe, telling me it was a bright spot in their day. It brought a whole new audience to all the perinatal mental health and OCD stuff. And for those following me because of the honest chat about darker themes, they suddenly had some comic relief. It was a brilliant merging of two worlds.

Some came for a giggle and learnt about maternal mental health. Some wanted to feel less alone in their struggles and smiled at a joke. Some just liked Josie from *Fresh Meat*. But they all stayed and this beautifully eclectic but accepting community was born.

And I laughed. I could laugh again. The sound had been so foreign to my own ears for such a long time. The hollowness was gone, too. I was honest to God belly-laughing because someone wrote to me: *What's the difference between a fanny and a fridge? A fridge doesn't fart when you take the meat out.* Or: *How do you think the unthinkable? With an itheberg!* Ridiculous. Ludicrous. But it felt like I could breathe again or a little easier, if only for a moment, and so it continued. And it felt like a move away from just feeling like an object of sympathy or eye-rolling. I was putting something else out there, which meant that maybe one day I wouldn't just be that girl with OCD who used to be on the telly.

I could be fun again. Have fun again. That side of me had been smothered for so long, I genuinely believed it had expired. But it hadn't, there was a pulse and signs of life. Just like all those years before when we had sat in that scan room, the little rabbit had been there all along.

Forty-five videos later and still counting, here are some of my favourites:

What's ET short for? He's only got little legs.

www.conjunctivitis.com – that's a site for sore eyes.

Did you see my joke about my chiropractor problems? It was about a weak back.

I've been ripped off. I paid a carpenter to make a double bed and he's done a bunk.

Time flies like an arrow. Fruit flies like a banana.

And my favourite . . .

What's green and smells of pork? Kermit's fingers.

Turns out laughter really is the best medicine.

9

The Real Afterbirth

(Or Kimfluencing My Brain™)

For the better part of two and a half years I lived in two realities. It was a bit like Keanu Reeves seeing into the Matrix. I knew what was really out there, but no one else seemed to believe me, so I'd comply and play my part in this charade and stick to the script. Yes, I'll have a coffee. I'm sorry? Oh, he's two years old now. Yes, it is a lovely age. Yes, it does go so fast. Another baby? Um, not sure, maybe. I'll miss it when he's older? If you say so.

I'd dipped my toe into being more honest. Not just with medical professionals but friends and family and eventually, the Internet. Now, somewhere in the midst of all this mental turmoil and sleepless nights, I ludicrously decided to go one step further. I decided to start a Substack. I'd only gone on Instagram to get free dungarees, remember (to this day, not a sausage).

I remember it clearly: it was 3am; I was on the floor leaning against my son's cot bars while he slept. Maybe I could write mini articles on unspoken parts of perinatal mental health, I thought. Things I would have loved to have read when I was feverishly googling to find some answers.

Hmmm, what should I call the Substack? In my family there's a long-running joke about how bad at influencing on Instagram I am. I'm not cool or chic or always put together, so there's little chance I'd have any influence over anyone. I decided to lean into this. I wasn't an influencer; I was a Kimfluencer. Crying laughing emoji. How about Kimfluencing My Brain as the title? That was sort of what I was doing. Shit, that was a terrible title. What did it even mean? Oh well, it was three in the morning and I didn't care anymore. Fine then, that would do. Did I want to add a podcast option before I pressed launch? Again, why the hell not? Everyone else had a podcast these days. But I decided I'd do things differently. I'd differentiate mine by having no edits, no scheduled delivery and absolutely no production value whatsoever. Just me, a tiny mic and my phone. What a classy piece of social media content this would be.

I ended up writing blogs and recording podcast episodes on everything from feeling like I would never get better to learning more about how my brain works. With such heavy-hitting titles as 'Angus, Thongs and Perfect Reunions' and 'Am I A Neurodivergent Ken Barlow?', I was sure a Pulitzer was in the post.

One editorial I put up, which was both the most necessary thing I've ever done and possibly the final nail in my career coffin, was called 'I Can't Say This Out Loud Yet'. It was a list you could print out (if you're old-school), or else just have on your phone to show to your doctor, health visitor or midwife (like a normal person). I really struggled with vocalising my symptoms and the content of my deeply upsetting thoughts. Saying it made it too real. Although I will say the content of the thoughts doesn't matter – I know I thought it did, and I thought mine were worse than anyone else's but it was my reaction to them that became the

THE REAL AFTERBIRTH

problem. Even now, sometimes I stand in a room alone and say my worry out loud. It never fails to sound ridiculous. Voicing it takes away its power. It just never seems to hold up outside of my mind, out in the real world.

Anyway, here is an extract:

Can't bring yourself to say the words? Then highlight what you're experiencing to show a health professional.

- I am having unrelenting, terrifying thoughts and images that I might be a danger to my baby.
- I'm having unrelenting, terrifying thoughts and images of a violent or sexual nature about harm coming to my baby.
- I'm in a constant state of 'Flight, Fright or Freeze'.
- I'm worried that I might 'snap' and hurt my baby.
- I do everything I can to protect my baby from myself.
- I'm constantly seeing a few seconds into the future with the most awful consequences.
- I'm hyperaware and vigilant ALL of the time. I can't switch it off.
- My love and protection instincts for my baby feel corrupted and sinister.
- I can't think clearly.
- I don't know what I'm feeling anymore.
- I feel everything too much.
- I need help but I don't know if I can be helped.
- I fear that every tiny decision I make regarding my baby is wrong.
- I fear my baby will die and it will be my fault.
- I fear my baby will get hurt and it will be my fault.
- I fear being left alone with my baby although I would

never hurt them, but I just can't be certain.
- I fear doing basic things for my baby e.g. nappy changes, breast-feeding or bathing in case I do something inappropriate by accident.
- I think about these terrible things so much I worry that it's because I want them and I have to keep checking I don't enjoy it.
- I truly believe I could be a monster and need to keep checking I'm not.
- These things take up much of my day and night.

You are not alone.

★

I had sleepless nights and nail-biting, stomach-churning days after posting this. But do you know what happened? People used it to get help. Suck it, OCD! I wasn't the worst of the worst. I wasn't beyond the pale. I was just a woman who'd had a traumatic birth, and whose brain was overreacting in exactly the same way it had my entire life.

Every single day for nearly two years I woke up with a crushing dread and a hope so dwindled, I was essentially surviving on embers. My first thought, without fail, was to check if the bad thoughts had gone. But by doing this simple act, I had already lost the battle for that day.

I'd checked therefore I'd thought. Descartes, eat your heart out. And I was tired. Very, very tired. I'd tried everything. I'd engaged with ERP but nothing seemed to be breaking through. However, I would soon acknowledge that while ardently, almost obsessively (funny that) and actively *exposing* myself to everything that I was afraid of, I hadn't been addressing the second part of the treatment – *response prevention*. I'd just held my baby and stared at him, willing the intrusive thoughts away, pushing through the intense anxiety to get to the other side. The promised land of recovery, where I could be normal again and my day would revolve around something – anything – else.

My brain thought it was helping me, protecting me. I was trying to disprove a negative. I needed to know – beyond a shadow of a doubt – that I would never, ever hurt or even think about hurting anyone. Ever. Once I knew this, I could just move on. Get on with my life. But hang on while I just checked one more time . . .

My brain needed some kindness. So, do you know what I did?

I stopped actively hating my brain and by extension, myself. The new rule was *'give yourself a break'*.

With all things in life, there needs to be balance and moderation. So while these days, I try not to beat myself up constantly and, if I need time to myself or feel a certain way that day, then that's okay, I also try to have some discipline. Just because the world is sometimes too loud and too much for me and I want to cover my head with the duvet and sleep until it quiets down again, doesn't mean I can, or should. So, the other half of the rule became ' . . . *but don't let yourself off the hook*'. Know when to ease off and when to push yourself. Like everything else, this takes time and practice. Being an adult is a nightmare. But not when my son looks at me like I hung the moon. Not when he giggles at me or, even better, tries to make *me* laugh. Or when he discovers something interesting and new that blows his tiny, extraordinary mind. Or cuddles up to me just because he wants to. Then, it's hard to find that it wasn't all worth it. And believe me when I sincerely express to you that I don't say that lightly. And going to the supermarket with him is one of my favourite things in the world now. We giggle together and play and hug and kiss and he's my little guy, just like I always wanted.

People often ask when I started to feel like myself again. The truth is, I don't. Learning I can never go back to how things were before frees me. There is a new me and she is here to stay. Let's makes her a good 'un. Then I'm asked when I started to feel better. I know what they want to hear, because it's exactly what I wanted to hear when I was back in those post-partum trenches. We want to hear it's instant – you wake up one day and it's all gone. You want to be told there's a silver bullet. A magic pill – take this and you'll be right as rain. Ironically, the day I stopped wishing for that was one of the turning points of my recovery. Again, everything takes time, and I know how frustratingly unfair that feels.

A lot of people ask me if I'm on medication and which kind helps the best (read: quickest). I always answer that I do take medication but never give specifics and never, ever recommend a particular kind. Firstly, because I have zero qualifications to safely do so, and secondly, because what works for me might not work for you and vice versa. The medication rollercoaster feels more like plummeting drops than steady rises but once you do find the right medication at the right dose, it can significantly help to even you out. I know it gives me breathing space, time to get my head above water so I can concentrate on using what I've learned in therapy instead of just trying to survive.

Journalling and breathing exercises have their place, but they

THE REAL AFTERBIRTH

were fucking useless to me in the early days when I was plagued mercilessly by intrusive thoughts, images and urges, and had no idea what OCD really was. One type of medication made me deeply suicidal; others had too many side effects (rapid weight gain, headaches, shakiness and sleeplessness, to name but a few). My doctor implored me to stick with a medication for six to eight weeks to allow it time to work. When it became obvious that it wasn't right for me, I then had to wean myself off it slowly and the withdrawal seemed liked a cruel dessert. My feet felt as though rigor mortis had set in but simultaneously like they were curling up the wrong way like the witch from *The Wizard of Oz* after she's squashed by Dorothy's house. It was excruciating and in my muddled mind felt like a physical manifestation of all the nastiness going on in my head. I would then start a new course of a different medication and desperately hope it would be The One.

I did get onto an even keel, which allowed me to gradually calm my anxiety at the thoughts and resist my compulsions, like rumination or mental self-punishment. The frequency of the intrusive thoughts began to drop and, slowly, things started to shift, albeit at what felt like a glacial pace.

But honestly, hand on heart, when did I start to recover? It was when I began to forgive myself – but that process wouldn't start until nearly two years postpartum. I hated myself for such a long time for becoming ill in the first place. I berated myself for thinking such terrible things. I was unceasingly unkind and callous to myself because I truly bought into the narrative that I deserved all that animosity and more. But how could I heal when I didn't really believe I was worthy of healing? The recovery started small: washing – and then, unbelievably, drying my hair; taking a thirty-minute walk by myself for a time out, laughing out loud at something on TV.

There was one more thing I did, which seems so innocuous and stupid as to be inconsequential, but which really helped me turn a corner. I love seasonal holidays – I always go all out – and yet any joy I usually felt at Christmas, Halloween and birthdays had been snuffed out over those first couple of years of motherhood. One day while out and about with the pram, looking around the shops on my local high street, I saw this hideous bright-orange sweatshirt with a black Jack-o'-Lantern face on it. It was £7, and instead of walking by or browsing and then putting it back – because fun wasn't for people like me – I bought it. My son had a similar jumper, and I dared to dream that those cute happy snap moments of matching outfits could be for us, too. Tiny to the outside world but a seismic moment of investing in a possible future happiness for me. A bud of possibility began to unfurl inside me, that maybe I was allowed to *enjoy* things again. That had been an alien concept to me for a very, very long time.

Trying to recover from OCD by not doing compulsions (for me, ruminating, rebuking myself, body-checking, excessively monitoring my baby, tensing my body to remain vigilant, clicking, head shaking, counting) is a bit like trying to become a millionaire one penny at a time. It's interminable and at times feels impossible but gently, under the radar, each time you resist and, more importantly, don't beat yourself up if you do slip up, your pile of pennies begins to grow. Suddenly your day isn't taken up by just that 'thing'. Other parts of your life come back into focus, and you begin to take pleasure in the little things again. You push yourself out of the small world you've limited yourself to.

THE REAL AFTERBIRTH

Maybe it's lunch with a friend, perhaps it's going to a party, or even having a massage. Ludicrously self-indulgent, I know, but I've always had a crappy, weak back and a really firm Thai massage is my guilty pleasure. The first time I went for one – maybe a year post-baby – after being physically tense and wrung out for all that time, I cried. I wasn't sobbing, but a little tear slipped out and was quickly absorbed by the tissue paper on the massage bed. The masseuse didn't even notice. But the idea of allowing someone to touch me and take care of me, of allowing myself to feel better, to have someone physically loosen my poor, taut muscles, which hadn't relaxed since that first day in the hospital all that time ago, when they'd wheeled my baby away and left me all alone to wait in a cold, unfeeling room. It was breathtaking.

It was at this point that all the joy and excitement and sheer love started to fill my life again and where not one single second with my glorious son was taken for granted. Not even now when he screams at me that shampoo suds are blinding his eyes and whimpers for a towel like a Victorian invalid, only to then repeatedly ask for five more minutes in the bath. Do I get stressed when he's screeching, the dog is barking, the telly is on somewhere way too loud, and I must remember to do fifty things by tomorrow lunchtime? Of course I do. I'd love to tell you that when you recover and gain a sense of control over your OCD, that life is easy from here on out. That it's all water off a duck's back. But it's not and that's okay.

However, things only got better (if you don't count the huge number of blips and dips – remember, recovery isn't linear). I slowly but surely reconnected with the world. I was honest about my mental health struggles and didn't try to hide out of shame any longer. To anyone. I went on to different jobs, learnt to just *be* with my son – no OCD strings attached – and trivial things made me smile once again. One day, I realised I was looking forward to watching a film with my husband and the baby later in the evening and maybe ordering a pizza. So simple, no fanfare. But I wasn't riddled with fear and doubt, and there was the possibility of it just 'being a nice time'. Nothing more, nothing less. Heavenly to my saturated mind that had been living in that hellscape forever and a day.

I also found listening to true crime podcasts a really useful tool in my recovery arsenal. At first, I wouldn't be able to get past imagining that I'd done all the terrible things being narrated to me but slowly, as I pushed through and persevered, the anxiety subsided. I've always been fascinated by crime (see: Agatha Christie hyperfixation), and once I was no longer scared of the unknown, I could simply listen and engage with the interesting story being told instead of me inserting myself into it. The same with true crime documentaries on Netflix. My natural inclination was to avoid them, not trigger myself with the scary content, but this was ultimately not helpful in showing my mind that it was okay. Nothing to do with us, brain. No emergency response required. And so now, I'm something of a connoisseur of the genre because it no longer bothers me.

In summer 2025, to add another acronym to my CV, I was diagnosed with autism and ADHD (or AuDHD in neurodiverse slang). I cried happy tears and finally felt that instant release of a huge weight being lifted off my shoulders, the one that I'd longed to feel all through that postpartum time. I think as an autistic person, the idea of responsibility has always been a big part of my life. If I'm told to do something and I follow the

THE REAL AFTERBIRTH

rules, then even when things go tits up, it can't all be my fault when generally a lot of things feel like they are. I've always taken responsibility for things that have nothing to do with me. Someone can't afford to go somewhere – I'll pay, even when I can't afford it. There's a bad atmosphere in the room – I must be overly jovial and fix it. So, when an amazing doctor – a psychologist who listened to me, carried out intensive diagnostic testing and dived into my entire life from birth to nearly forty and came to the clinical conclusion that I had an autistic brain with Attention Deficit Hyperactivity Disorder, it was the biggest 'it's not your fault' I'd ever felt.

I've lived my entire life as a neurotypical person trying to fit in. It's not even a square peg in a round hole; it's more an oval peg in a round hole – it looks like it should fit but somehow never quite aligns. You can hammer it into place but after each knock, the peg looks a little worse for wear. After forty years of knocks, that poor peg is bruised and more out of shape than ever. There are ways I think and things I do that I have, subconsciously or not, tried to remedy my entire life. It's why snippets of conversations would play over and over for days or weeks, sometimes years at a time. Why my memory is both incredible and foggy. I can spot and recall details that seem to slide by everyone else but when I try to complete a simple task – like putting clean laundry away – it becomes an insurmountable blur. I feel defeated so quickly, angry with myself and confused as to what I'm meant to be doing. A task-blindness takes over. You may wonder how one writes a whole book with that kind of a brain, and the answer is that I currently have nine different chapters all open on my laptop and haven't finished one of them. I bounce between them as new ideas occur, or I can't think where to go next.

My brain feels like I'm watching three televisions sets at the same time. Each one is playing a different TV show at assorted volumes and varying speeds. Sometimes they sync up, often they don't, and it's hard for me to decide where my attention should be. It's as exhausting as it sounds. So, while my husband will get frustrated that I've become distracted while he's talking to me, I'm actually tuning in to another programme for a few moments. If I'm having a particularly tough time, there will be a couple of different radio stations playing in the background too. When I was extremely poorly, it was all of the above but it felt as if I was also tied to a chair in the middle of a locked room and couldn't reach the TVs or radios to switch them off while yelling for someone to come and help – but I couldn't be heard because a stuck record player was spinning a vinyl of horror screams over and over. Maybe now you can see why I sometimes have to ask, 'What did you just say?'

In Greek mythology, when Pandora's box was opened, she released all the evils of the world but the one thing that remained inside was hope. My box, so to speak, had been empty for a long time. I had never been so devoid of hope in all my life. I'd had hard times – depressive episodes, spirals and huge anxiety – but there was always something to give me a grain of hope. A hug, my favourite film, a sweet snack, tiny bumps of endorphins. But suddenly, there was nothing, and I scraped around in the dirt looking for so long. An existence without hope is one of the scariest things I've ever faced. For the better part of two and a half years, I was adrift, treading water in a vast, open ocean, unable to reach any of the lifelines that were haphazardly thrown my way. The only options were to keep swimming against the tide, stop and let the water swallow me whole, or keep looking for a lifeboat to come along and scoop me out.

It was only when I realised there was a secret fourth option that my thinking slowly morphed. I could lie on my back, look up at the sky and allow the waves to slowly bring me back to shore.

There's a leaflet I once saw at Barry Island, produced by the RNLI. It was about how to stop yourself panicking and making the situation worse if you fall into deep water. It was called Float to Live, and the tagline was 'Fight your instinct, not the water'. They used the acronym F.L.O.A.T. to remind you what to do:

Fight against your instinct to panic or swim harder.

Lean back in the water to keep your airway clear.

Open yourself up – extend your arms and legs and push your stomach up.

Actions – *GENTLY* move your arms and feet to help you float.

Time – in 60–90 seconds you'll be able to control your breathing.

I think OCD charities should adopt the same slogan – it's the only advice that rings true. By letting the fake urgency that your OCD is driving down onto you pass, you let the panic subside and then you're back in the driving seat. It's minimal but so incredibly powerful after riding shotgun in your own life for so long.

Now, when I get what I call 'hot neck' – a wave of sensory overload – I need a break like everyone else, but I also take a moment to appreciate that I'm no longer fighting on two fronts. My mind is clearer and more forgiving. I don't beat myself up when things feel too much. I don't berate myself for not always having all the parenting answers. I'll work it out, one thing at a time. I'm no longer living in a dual reality and there's a sense of peace within me now that I don't think I'll ever take for granted.

*

My greatest fear during those darker days was that my bond with my son was being irretrievably broken. That I'd scuppered his early development by being so unwell and that he would always *know*, somehow, that I had found those initial years too difficult. He would innately think less of me. In fact, it's turned out to be almost the exact opposite. Our relationship is stronger for everything we've been through together. I showed up every day when, frankly, all I wanted to do was curl up under a rock and die like a wretched little Granny Grey, which is testament to how extraordinary he is – and how strong our connection is. We are tactile and affectionate and that warms me rather than fills me with panic or dread. Our faces both light up when we see each other and that's all I could ever ask for. He makes me laugh, deep belly laughs and each one feels even more special because I know the alternative.

My OCD chirps up whenever it can to worry me, but pushing through with a metaphorical shrug isn't feeding the beast and it soon fizzles away. OCD craves certainty, a certainty you can never fully reach. How sure is sure? Learning to live in the maybe, to doggy paddle in the grey, is one of the greatest challenges you can face with this condition, but equally it will earn you the quickest rewards. Of course, you have to ensure your shrug doesn't become a physical compulsion, like I had with clicking my fingers or shaking my head to neutralise the thoughts. Again, OCD is a tricky fucker and can be sneaky. You're not willing the thoughts away. You're lying on your back and bathing in them until the urgency passes and the stakes aren't quite so high. Your own private lagoon of self-acceptance.

Learning that sometimes doing nothing – not fighting my thoughts, not repeating punishing compulsions, not thinking that spending every minute criticising every aspect of myself is the best way to keep everyone safe – has been my greatest discovery. I let the thoughts just be there. I tried not to judge them, fix them, replace them or neutralise them but live my life anyway. So I would meet a friend for coffee even if I didn't hear a word they said; go to a family dinner and linger like an outsider – the ghost at the feast – or pop to the cinema to watch some blockbuster superhero sequel, even if I cried into my popcorn all the way through. And slowly, glimmers of hope began to return. A little oxytocin kicked in at buying a new dress, I'd look forward to a social event in a week or so that could be – dare I say it – fun. A chuckle at a sitcom here, a productive work event there. And soon I was swimming through my hard-won pennies like Scrooge McDuck.

The more I've learnt about myself, my brain and my OCD, the easier it has been to decipher between an OCD thought and a perfectly natural question. I find that if there is a time pressure exerted – for example, touch that lamppost right now or something bad will happen – then it's usually OCD. If you can say to yourself, I have this work dilemma or relationship issue, but I will focus on it in ten minutes' time, I find it to be a 'real-world' problem – real-world problems will still be there in ten minutes if you haven't clicked your fingers. I now practise sitting in the anxiety and still being okay every chance I get. I count in my head a lot. I prefer multiples of five or ten, so a really low-level exercise is to put the TV volume on seventeen and leave it. Even now, thinking about it, there's a slight rumble under my skin telling me that's not okay. So, I ride the tiny wave – more boogie-boarding than pro-surfing – and then I'll be more capable when the next tsunami hits. Or when I'm picking things up and I MUST pick up ten items at a time, I deliberately only fetch nine and push through the 'need' to correct it. These seem like small steps, but when a bigger OCD episode hits, you'd be amazed how much you've rewired your brain and suddenly, your immediate response of 'quick, react now', is swiftly followed by a 'but if you don't, that's okay too'.

The main difference I feel now, a few years on, is that the thoughts haven't changed but they are far less frequent. And my bounce-back time after having a setback is far quicker too. Having a bad day doesn't have to mean having a bad week or month. It can just be that: a crappy day where things are affecting me more than usual. That used to mean everything was ruined. I'd given in to a compulsion? That's the day gone. Two in a row? Forget it. I may as well hibernate. Everything inside my mind is always so black and white. It's perfect or it's ruined. But real life seldom adheres to those rules. I'll say it again: recovery isn't linear. The line on the graph doesn't just travel in a smooth upward trajectory; it will look more like a cardiogram with peaks and troughs, and that's okay. The general direction is up, even when it doesn't feel like it.

★

One thing that surprises me, more than it should, is the need for people to ask, 'When are you having another baby?' During that first eighteen months after giving birth, the idea of getting pregnant again was my ultimate nightmare. I feared it would break me in a way that I wouldn't be able to come back from. That badly pieced-back-together vase would crumble into dust. I was barely making it through this, and people wanted me to put myself through it again? Why? Because my family wasn't complete?

My family does feel incomplete sometimes. I never expected to only have one child. I always imagined my future filled with little siblings bickering and protecting each other. A full house. But in other ways our little family of three is everything and feels more than whole.

The thing that people don't warn you about when you only have one child is that you're sometimes dubbed as selfish. You must like all that disposable income too much; you don't want to be inconvenienced by going through that baby phase again. You're too worried about your body. Well, yeah, people haven't stopped commenting on my body my whole life. I was too thin, gangly, lanky, then I was too big – put on some timber, chubby. Then I was pregnant and everyone – Covid permitting – thought they could touch me and give me unsolicited advice.

My morning sickness was so acute that I lost a lot of weight. Then when my pregnancy advanced and I picked up, I ate better than I ever had. Good, green, folic-filled vegetables. Bananas were eaten on long, invigorating hikes with Bob. Boiled eggs were gobbled as a great protein snack. We had been through so much to get there that I wanted the baby to be as healthy and supported as possible – pessaries in the wrong orifice notwithstanding. After the birth, I dropped so much weight that I was back in normal jeans within a month. Everyone thought this was marvellous. I was trying to knit my mind back together, but I was dropping stitches faster than I could count. Still, as long as I was sufficiently slim enough to warrant some sort of invisible societal award, that's all that counted. As I moved through the illness, I punished myself by not looking after my health. I started to put weight on. This, I discovered, was bad – if people's cruel comments were anything to go by. But now I was confused. I felt better as I navigated recovery and could actually tolerate eating, but people were saying I looked 'amazing' before when I was gaunt and suicidal. People are so weird.

So, now I'm better and on a more steady footing, I'm selfish for not wanting to go back and do it all again? And remember, it's not a case of us just not using protection and seeing what happens. It means going back to the start of IVF – we'd have to go private, as we no longer qualify for free treatment – and work hasn't been prolific enough for us to afford God knows however many rounds and cycles. Even if I put myself through the rigorous hormonal regime and invasive scans again, I may not get pregnant. I may not *stay* pregnant. If I did, there would be the birth, and although it would be under normal, not pandemic, conditions, my faith in hospitals and medical professionals has been eroded to nought.

And if I safely carry and deliver a beautiful healthy baby, what then? That's when my troubles started last time. What if I become ill again? It's a 'what if' worth pursuing, for once – I told you you'd start to be able to tell the difference. But as I keep improving and the idea of becoming pregnant again doesn't scare the ever-loving shit out of me, I know I'm starting to amble down an unhealthy path. What if this time I could do it better? What if I could have a baby and not lose my mind? I could enjoy things and live my life. My son would have a little brother or sister, and I wouldn't be so useless and selfish. But that's a sneaky back-door OCD compulsion, trying to make me correct or fix something I can't.

I sometimes feel a powerful surge of broodiness that I thought I would never feel again. It's like biology has reared its horny little head and realised that the heat, almost literally, is on. This body needs to reproduce and do it fast! We're running out of time! It's like conceiving around forty is one big episode of *Ninja Warrior*. We have talked about it; recently, we even made an appointment to see a fertility doctor. They needed to cancel; we never rearranged. But the truth is we don't need it. Yes, there's a world where I have another baby and it's how it's 'supposed' to be. I'm not left alone for days on end on a lonely hospital ward, cut off from my family and allowed to almost wither on the NHS waiting-list vine. A life where having a second child is glorious, where I enjoy late-night feeds and don't feel like my skin is crawling every time I want to snuggle with my own newborn. But the fact I can even consider this a possibility is the real miracle. The honest truth is we just don't know. If I were to suddenly discover I was pregnant, I think we would genuinely be over the moon. We know so much more now. I gave birth as an undiagnosed autistic woman with chronic OCD during a pandemic and I survived it. Things *have* to be easier second time round. But there's a big difference between naturally falling pregnant and putting yourself through expensive and exacting IVF rounds that might yield nothing but more heartache. Again, I would just be trying to correct something that didn't need fixing.

But what of that fourth embryo, I hear you cry! We don't know, she winces in reply. One day, in the middle of my OCD post-partum black hole, I received a letter from the fertility clinic informing us our year of free storage was up and to pick a payment plan. I have no idea where that letter went and at the time didn't have the bandwidth to entertain such nonsense as having another baby. I was just trying to make it to twelve o'clock that day. We always called the fourth embryo Danny DeVito - specifically referring to his character from the movie *Twins* due to my misunderstanding of the 'quality' of an embryo. Was a 'good quality' embryo a Schwarzenegger, then? Turns out, no. I will try to track you down, dearest Danny, but I fear you may have perished on a windowsill somewhere in Heath Hospital, having never achieved your full potential. But maybe we'll meet again. Don't know where, don't know when.

Today, I press on with Kimfluencing My Brain, God love me. I'm more candid on Instagram about what real OCD, and in particular perinatal OCD, looks like. I often write the hashtag: #smashthestigma. Nice bit of virtue signalling there, but what do I mean? I mean: say the bad thing out loud and see that your life doesn't come crashing down around you. In fact, you'll find you give others the courage to say 'me too'. They'll open up, allowing you to become even braver. Will there be people who don't understand? Of course, but please believe me when I tell you they are few and far between. I've not met a parent yet who doesn't feel some relief at leaning into a conversation about the toll trying to be a good mum or dad takes. It doesn't mean we don't love our kids with every fibre of our being or wish for a different life; it's just a vent. Would I die for my son? Without hesitation. But what he actually needs is for me to *live* for him. To try to be better, healthier, the truest version of me and not harangue myself

THE REAL AFTERBIRTH

when I sometimes fall short. To show him how to be a human being. Perfectly imperfect – foibles, failures, gifts and triumphs and all the mundanity in between.

That's why I actively stop myself from feeling the intense mum-guilt I felt when I had to work. When I'm not working, I'm with my son and husband, non-stop. When I get the opportunity to do what I love, I grab it with both hands because it's important that my son sees a fully rounded-out human being who can be different things at the same time. I can be a silly playmate for him, then a stern mam. I can be affectionate with my husband while telling him he's doing my head in. I can be a creative, out-in-the-world person and still come home to nestle into our little bubble there. I can shoot TV shows, write books and scripts, chat about films on a podcast, visit different parts of the bubble and all through a job I love. Not bad for a girl from a tiny village in the Valleys. I can also be happy and frustrated and tired and imaginative and kind and selfish, all at the same time. And so can you. We are a multitude, and our brains can lie to us. If I had listened to my brain all those years ago in that bitterly cold, barren woodland, I would have broken my dad's heart. I would have shattered my soulmate, and I would never have spent these last few years of cuddling, joking and giggling with my golden-haired, giant-hearted boy.

My son and I are two peas in a pod. I see so much of myself in him, and while after his birth that thought would have terrified me because I wanted to keep him safe and protected, not tainted by my warped brain, now it makes me smile. He makes me smile. Even on my worst days, he's made me smile. I see patterns of behaviour in him that I recognise and feel so heartened that as he grows up, he will view neurodiversity and thinking differently as not just a curse, but also a gift. If you can reframe your thinking and not let your own brain terrify you, then the whole world can suddenly open up for you. I hope that the whole world will continue to open up for him because he is surrounded by people who understand and celebrate who he is. It takes time to get there, and you have to start small. Remember how I said that an embryo is a tenth of the size of a full stop? Smaller than that. But eventually the glimmers start to expand into the brightest light.

Find the glimmers. They are there if you just dare to look up.

I wouldn't change my little boy for the world and while I wish I hadn't been so unbearably ill for so long, it wasn't my fault.

Fuck, it's taken years to get to this. It's not my fault. It's not your fault either.

I hope in time you'll be able to see that too. Because, and I mean this in the kindest way possible, you're just not *that* original. You're not the first person to think something and you certainly won't be the last, even when your brain tries to convince you otherwise.

Take it from me. Happy to be totally unoriginal.

THE END
(And I only used the word 'journey' once)

Epilogue

I'd wanted to write a book for a very long time, even before I really had anything to write a book about. To me, it was the ultimate in intellectual swagger, patience and dedication. To sit at a desk, in a proper chair and write a worthy tome, taking time now and then to sip freshly brewed coffee and survey beautiful gardens out of my window.

I bought a chair for this book. It's from TK Maxx. It was £99. A pale-pink, mid-century office chair. It has arms and everything. Much like the naff pumpkin jumper from years ago, it was an investment in my willingness to do something positive. Something for me. To look forward, while reflecting, and become a writer.

Have I sat in that chair once to write a word of this? Have I fuck. I've written this book lying in bed, sitting in the garden, at the kitchen table and curled up on the couch. I've written it in every conceivable position the human body is able to loll in for hours at a time. A foot up on a radiator, a pillow under my lower back, a yoga twist while I slowly shift away from the creeping direct sunlight. I've been a one-woman Kama Sutra, transcribing this book into my bashed-about green laptop. But

I can thank my AuDHD hypermobility for that. Every now and then my husband pokes his head in, asking me if I've backed it up. I tell him yes (I haven't) and then will randomly email myself a chapter in case I drop my computer and lose the whole thing. Rewrites were done in my local coffee shop from open to close because it's the only way I could remove distractions.

I tell you this as it's one of the most important lessons I've learned. It's two-fold really. Primarily, there is no right way to do everything. Or to be. Or to think and feel. I've thought for much of my life that I'm always doing things the *wrong* way. I'm feeling too much about this or paying too little attention to that. Writers are proper people who sit at desks, using huge reference books while capturing their well-thought-out stories, at properly scheduled times. Well, not this writer!

The second constituent part to the life lesson is learning not to care. Or, at least, so much it permeates every area of your life. I don't feel an ounce of guilt about not using that chair. Years ago, I would have. I would have dithered over buying it, then tried to stick to a strict timetable of how and when to write the book that I thought other people wanted me to write. I almost certainly wouldn't have told you about my first postpartum poo, but they are the elements that make up who I really am. These days I'm consciously not trying to fit a mould that simply won't contain me. I want to do things how I want to do them, when I want to do them, and I no longer beat myself up about that.

I also realised before tapping a single key that if I wasn't going to be honest in this book, there was no point. If you'd have wanted a 'How To', you'd have read a book by some qualified paediatrician or psychologist. If you'd wanted a beautiful photo book for your coffee table where I'm in a crisp

EPILOGUE

white, flowing dress surrounded by a carefully curated minimalist living room, everything pristine and shining, a smiley baby in one arm, wildflowers in the other, again, you'd have bought a different book. I hope you wanted to read this book because it's real. Am I scared I've gone too far? Been too dark and said too much? Yes. That OCD claw is hooked into the back of my hot neck and is goading me to digitally highlight every word and delete it. That's safer. But does it help anyone? Does how we deal with this stuff as a society change? No.

I wanted to write my story – this book – to show not only you but also myself that it's all okay. That we don't have to love every minute, we don't even have to like it. There is no script for life. My body and brain have thrown up things during fertility, pregnancy, birth and the proceeding years that I never could have predicted. And I hated myself for such a long time for not being like everybody else. But there is no 'everybody else'. There's just you and your set of circumstances and doing your best on that day. Which on some days can be simply brushing your teeth. Every now and then, you'll have a mum day where you're killing it. Once in a blue moon, you'll feel like you're in a shampoo commercial getting into the car for the school run, a little early after your child has been cute and charming all morning. Treasure it. Those moments are like hen's teeth.

We recently took our little boy for his first camping trip (huge disclaimer: my brother set the tent up, brought all the equipment and did all the boring bits, while I got to roast marshmallows over the fire, snuggle up with my son in the sleeping bags with a Paddington book and play hide and seek in the woods). At one point, I took him into the toilet block.

There was a woman brushing her teeth at the sinks. As I helped him to the loo, he happily chatted away, apropos nothing, about all the vegetables he loves to eat and the flowers and leaves he wants to pick. Getting him to eat vegetables is murder, although I concede he has a good appetite for fruit. His fruit budget is equal to that of the GDP of a small country. Apples, remember? Anyway, he was going on and on about how he adores tomatoes and runner beans and fresh corn, and it was all bullshit. But it occurred to me that if I were the woman outside the stall brushing my teeth, I would be thinking, 'Shit, she is *nailing* it.'

But it's only a snippet of the reality. She didn't see the huge temper tantrum ten minutes before and again half an hour afterwards, when he was bored of the river and wanted an ice-cream. I'm not saying that everything you see in real life or online is all fabricated – I'm not that much of a cynic – but I want you to know you're not alone. The more I learn about my neurodiverse brain, my autism, my ADHD and then my OCD on top of that, the more I have to keep reminding myself that it's okay to be me.

Acting is a lot like motherhood. Everyone is winging it and some are better than others at looking like they have it all. But let's not forget the financial aspect either. Behind that beautiful monochrome interior design and carefree 'mom life' on social media is a cleaner, a nanny, a make-up artist, a nail technician, a stylist, a driver, a personal trainer and a chef. You'd look like that too if you had an army of help. I know they say it takes a village but that's a pricey one. And I don't begrudge it. I'd love that. But pretending you have your shit together, as I found out, can be harmful to the self-confidence of mums who are just getting by.

EPILOGUE

Which is the norm, by the way. I know we can now see what's a #ad, but maybe we should enforce a #hadhelp rule so you're aware that this didn't all just happen. I see posts on Instagram of women doing their 5am run before waking up their compliant, darling children to serve them a home-made, nutritionally balanced breakfast while sharing daily affirmations and going on to the school run looking like they're about to shoot a teeth-whitening commercial. I'm sorry, what in the actual fuck? It can make you feel hugely lacking when your morning routine looks more like a time-blind, clothing malfunction during feeding time at the chimp enclosure. I barely get a bra on for school drop-off. #needhelp

In my business, you also become shrewd at spotting the good eggs. When someone I have worked with goes on to win a BAFTA or land a huge job, I'm so chuffed for them. It's great when good things happen to good people. Same in real life. Real women cheering on and supporting other women is genuinely one of the best feelings, but to do that, everyone has to be a little more honest. And a little less presented. My friendship with Jess works because, since we were eleven, we've never really tried to pretend with each other. The first thing one of us says is 'I haven't washed my hair in a week' or 'the kids had McDonald's for tea – I'm knackered'.

This book would have saved my life back in those dark, dark days when I felt so alone and such a burden that I'd convinced myself that the world would be a better place, and my family would have a better life, without me in it. So, my greatest wish is that if you've resonated with any part of my story – if you've had a single moment of 'that's me!' or 'oh my god, I did that' – then I'm happy to share every humiliating, embarrassing and shocking aspect of becoming a mother (hence sharing arse pessaries, dildo practice and lonely pooing), because I support you. And I hope you support me, too. One truth at a time; we can change the way an entire generation talks about perinatal mental health and what it means to be a mother today, where you're expected to climb the ladder, bounce back, practise self-care and be all things, to all people, all the time.

That's bullshit and now you know that someone else thinks that too.

And I still wear those giant pregnancy pants. No fucks given.

Acknowledgements

This book wouldn't have been possible without the incredible support and unwavering belief in me from Michelle Signore at Simon and Schuster. From our very first meeting, I was made to feel like my story was important, valid and deserved to be told. You never asked me to be anything other than who I was, or to write in any other way than from the heart and for that there are not enough thank yous in the world.

Thank you to Alison MacDonald, who helped to edit the book with such faith and compassion in what we were doing. And to Sophie Bradshaw for coming in and restructuring the book – especially the second half. It was so helpful for my foggy, ADHD-addled brain to see the bigger picture that much more clearly. Thank you to Maudisa King and Clare Wallis for making me clarify things I'd answered in my head but not on the page, thus making it better for the reader.

Thank you to my acting agent Ollie Azis, and his wonderful assistant, Lizzie Price, who never showed me anything other than complete understanding and compassion – that my well-being was more important than any job. From IVF through the long road to recovery, they were truly the best team to have my back.

To my husband – thank you for allowing me to 'go dark' for days at a time to write this. For looking after our son, for telling me that I could do it and for telling me that you were proud of me. I don't thank you for your notes, which I took *very* personally – as is my right as a wife.

Thank you to my little boy. My entire heart. Every time I looked up from the screen and wondered what the hell I was doing, I would take you in, and it would strengthen my resolve – how far we've come, how much we have to look forward to, and how I would walk through fire for you. But also, if you keep saying 'Mammy' eighty times in five minutes, I might scream – as is my right as a mother.

And to you, dear reader, who now knows the worst of me, but whom I hope doesn't think less of me. I hope I made you feel less alone. You've certainly done that for me.

Notes

Chapter 1: IVF

1 https://www.physio-pedia.com/Vaginismus

Chapter 5: Intrusive Thoughts

2 https://www.ocduk.org/ocd/types/
3 Cox J. L., Holden J. M. and Sagovsky R., 'Detection of postnatal depression: Development of the 10-item Edinburgh Postnatal Depression Scale', *British Journal of Psychiatry* 150 (1987), pp. 782–86.

Chapter 6: Dear Diary

4 Gemma Dunstan, 'Online abuse: "I found out my husband had indecent images"', *BBC News* (16 March 2021) at https://www.bbc.co.uk/news/uk-wales-56404743
5 Fiona Collardeau, Beth Corbyn, Jonathan S. Abramowitz *et al.*, 'Maternal unwanted and intrusive thoughts of infant-related harm, obsessive-compulsive disorder and depression in the perinatal period: study protocol', *BMC Psychiatry* 19 (2019), article 94.
6 Ibid.